Medical Case Studies (Consilia medica) of the Early Modern Period

Medical Case Studies (Consilia medica) of the Early Modern Period

Great Pox Documented

Bohdana Divišová

Translated by Frank A. Schultz

Routledge
Taylor & Francis Group
LONDON AND NEW YORK

First published in 2022 by Amsterdam University Press Ltd.

Published 2025 by Routledge
4 Park Square, Milton Park, Abingdon, Oxon OX14 4RN
605 Third Avenue, New York, NY 10158

Routledge is an imprint of the Taylor & Francis Group, an informa business

ISBN: 9789463723640 (hbk)
ISBN: 9781041182672 (pbk)
ISBN: 9781003699552 (ebk)
NUR 684

Cover illustration: Physicians surrounding a patient (from title page of Latin translation of Galen's works published by Frobenius in 1561)
© Library of Institute for History of Medicine and Foreign Languages, First Faculty of Medicine, Charles University

Cover design: Coördesign, Leiden

DOI: 10.5117/9789463723640

For Product Safety Concerns and Information please contact our EU representative:
GPSR@taylorandfrancis.com
Taylor & Francis Verlag GmbH, Kaufingerstraße 24, 80331 München, Germany

Table of Contents

1 Introduction

Abstract

The reader is introduced to the term "consilium," a written account of one specific case of a disease with advice regarding medical treatment. In the 16th century, consilia literature was a common component in the practices of many eminent physicians, and often served as a substitute for the "epistolae medicinales" genre. Today, consilia are unjustifiably neglected as a source of the history of medicine, even though they contain a lot of interesting information about the practices of elite physicians, their mutual communication, and patients. This has been documented through the study of consilia collections created by 15 physicians. Special attention has been paid to consilia written for patients suffering from the French disease or syphilis.

Keywords: syphilis, 16th century, medicine, consilia

"A glorious case!" This enthusiastic shout escaped the mouth of the founder of clinical education, Professor Giovanni Battista da Monte, at the bedside of a man with a decomposing face, afflicted by uncontrollable tremors and covered with horrifying ulcers.[1] This occurred in Padua in the year 1543 and was witnessed by medical students at the beginning of one of eight instruction sessions on the topic of the "French disease" at the municipal Hospital of St. Francis. Of course, we are not informed in detail regarding some of the circumstances surrounding this event, but the scene described is not entirely fictitious. The professor's commentary was captured by one of the medical students present, who evidently later provided this together with other commentaries to his colleague Johann Crato, who published them under the common Latin title "Consultationum medicarum opus" as a compilation of medical consultations. However, the individual cases

1 „Pulcherrimus casus!" Montanus, *Consultationum medicarum opus,* 867. Cons. CCCLXIII. Cura post morbum gallicum.

Divišová, Bohdana, *Medical Case Studies (Consilia medica) of the Early Modern Period.*
Taylor & Francis Group, 2022
doi: 10.5117/9789463723640_ch01

captured in this anthology do not bear the designation "consultatio" but are instead called "consilium." As will be demonstrated below, physicians during the early modern period viewed these terms as synonyms. In order to meet the objectives of this work however, it is necessary to differentiate these terms. Therefore, the genre of the 17th and 18th century will be called "consultation literature," while "consilia literature" will be reserved for the analogous genre of the 16th century.

Da Monte's lecture at the bedside of the syphilis patient is not a typical consilium, neither in the way we perceive it today, nor in what this word meant in the 16th century. At that time, a consilium above all represented a written account of one specific case of a disease with advice regarding medical treatment. This advice was usually requested by a physician, who had doubts regarding the treatment of a particular patient. The responding counsellor, usually a famous expert, usually never even saw his colleague's patient in person, which did not matter much considering the diagnostic capabilities of the times. This approach was still common in the early modern period and consilia literature, together with other analogous medical genres, became very popular.

In the course of the 16th century, the French disease also became very "popular."[2] It spread to all social classes of the population, including of course the highest classes from which the recipients of consilia usually came. Gaspar Torella (1452-1520), the personal physician of Pope Alexander VI. (the infamous Rodrigo Borgia), named the new disease "morbus curialis" due to its spreading at all courts of both the secular and ecclesiastical nobility, which was also done by other physicians.[3] As a disease with a chronic course and an unbelievable number of different symptoms and medical problems, lues was destined to become an ideal topic of a large number of consilia. During the peak of humanism, many erudite physicians created consilia some of which were gathered into collections and spread via printing. Although the popularity of this literature continued for at least the subsequent two centuries, the expert public knows relatively little about it.

We can only guess the reasons why consilia undeservedly remain outside the realm of expert interest. It is possible that consilia only aroused interest during the period of their development and establishment which occurred in about the 14th-15th centuries. As a widespread and entirely common genre, they are no longer so interesting. Lesser interest may also be attributed to

2 For historical reasons, which will be explained below, the terms French disease or the great pox will be used exclusively to designate this disease.

3 For details see Kümmel, "De morbis Aulicis," 18-9.

the current orientation of historians of medicine on "Patientengeschichte," which puts consilia at a disadvantage since the communication they capture usually takes place at the physician-to-physician level.

Another one of the reasons may be an antiquated methodological perspective of the history of medicine. Until relatively recent times, researchers in this area, often physicians themselves, exclusively focused on mapping the development of the achievements and scientific approaches of the "greatest benefaction of humanity" which have led to the current level of Western medicine.[4] The works of the top physicians connected with the creation of consilia were only studied for traces of the ideas that enabled the rapid development of European medicine in the 19th century. For understandable reasons, one cannot expect that practically oriented consilia would capture discussions about modern medical theories or descriptions of revolutionary anatomical discoveries.

However, this perspective of the history of medicine has been revised in the last half century. Researchers have stopped tracking "progressive" and condemning "backward" medical opinions and theories. Instead, they have started to show greater interest in the capture of the discourse for each particular level of the development of medicine and individual diseases.[5] This shift has turned the interest of historians of the early modern period towards expert genres based on autopsies and practical experience which were emphasized by the Humanists – "observationes, casus, consultationes, historiae, epistolae medicinales."[6] Especially here, we find information about the professional activities of a physician, his "bread and butter" as well as extraordinary cases.[7]

The gathering of consilia into collections documents the growing interest about individual cases with individual patients. The fashion of consilia and their compilation was doubtlessly influenced by a range of factors, for example: the fame of the physician, the prominent status of the patient, the adeptness with which the physician was able to demonstrate when selecting an interpretation of the disease, and the range of medical authorities that he was able to cite and apply. The application of these skills was then

4 For an explanation of the origin of this connection see Porter, *The Greatest Benefit*, 4.

5 For details about the development and historiography of the history of medicine e.g. Eckart and Jütte, *Medizingeschichte* or Černý, *Mor 1480-1730*, 13-26.

6 For details about these related forms of medical literature see chapter 3.2 of this work.

7 The latest and most complete work dealing with almost all areas of medicine is the work of the distinguished historian of medicine M. Stolberg. Unfortunately, it was not possible to use the results of his research for this study. The new findings would certainly significantly enrich this work. See Stolberg, *Gelehrte Medizin und ärztlicher Alltag*.

reciprocally beneficial to the physician's career and his self-promotion. However, the main reason for the popularity of collections of consilia was the fact that they could supply their readers, either beginning physicians or more often medical students, with a large number of examples of how eminent experts handled the most problematic part of Galenic medicine: the selection of the right medications for a patient with a specific physical constitution and suffering from a particular disease.

Consilia were intended exclusively for the small financially secure classes of society: members of the secular and ecclesiastical nobility, wealthy municipal officials, merchants, lawyers and to a lesser extent, the wives and children of these social classes. With a certain amount of methodological circumspection, one can obtain interesting information about the diseases from which they suffered, their dietary habits and lifestyles. When studying them however, one must keep in mind the main pitfall that could significantly affect any potential research and its findings. Above all with respect to retrospective diagnosis, one must not forget that the described symptoms were classified and interpreted in accordance with the level of medical science of the given period. Even today, this fact is often ignored and the details obtained tend to be identified with current diseases. The results can then be misleading because as the current work of historians of medicine shows, the capabilities of retrospective diagnosis are limited to a certain extent.[8] If we briefly focus on the diseases captured in the consilia, we find that wealthy groups of the population seem most of all to have suffered from the chronic symptoms of various diseases: headaches, overall weakness, problems with digestion, fevers, swelling, etc. This fact can however be explained by the character of the consilia as letters and capabilities, specifically the speed of communication at that time.[9]

Even when a consilium was addressed to a patient, there is no doubt that its deciphering and practical application were in the hands of a physician. Since the genre originated, the vast majority of consilia were written in Latin and could also contain bibliographic references or such detailed instructions that they would be incomprehensible to even an educated layman. And it is just these formulations and other indications or even random references, which the consulted physician used, that make it possible to determine a whole range

8 For details about the problems and capabilities of retrospective diagnosis see e.g. Arrizabalaga, "Problematizing Retrospective Diagnosis," 51-70; or Karenberg, "Retrospective Diagnosis," 140-45.

9 In early modern period consilia literature, the number of consilia concerning acute cases increased in number. However, these are mostly supplementary records and thus not "real" consilia.

of facts not only about the physician himself, but also reveal the complexity of the professional hierarchy, social dynamics and relationships between individual and even groups of physicians – representatives of one faculty, one "collegium medicorum" (physicians' guild) or one specific city. Consilia also include references to representatives of other professions involved in the therapeutic process – surgeons, midwives, pharmacists, but most of all hacks against whom the patient was often warned in consilia. Thanks to this, we can also learn about the social and professional diversity of people involved in the treatment of the patient. Precisely the last-named group, which physicians usually disparagingly called "empirici, medicastri, agyrtae," actively expanded its activities in the initial stage of the French disease.

The outbreak of the French "plague" (lues) caused a range of controversies, debates and of course even fear among contemporaries. The first reactions consisted of a mix of practical, speculative and moral explanations of the disease referring to both natural processes as well as moral failure and the potential violation of various societal taboos. In the first years following the outbreak of the epidemic, this new disease attracted the attention of a large part of the scientific medical community. From the middle of the 16th century, when it changed from an epidemic to an endemic disease, it somewhat lost its touch of novelty and the reactions of physicians became more stable. How did the approach of physicians to syphilis patients change between the end of the 15th century and the beginning of the 17th century? What was the attitude of the top university-educated medical experts towards the treatment of a disease that was viewed as treatable and (not only) sexually transmittable? Did the often-proclaimed approach to this disease as a stigma already manifest itself during this period? Although a large number of theoretical medical monographs and treatises were written about the French disease in the course of the 16th century, consilia offer the best opportunity to capture how elite physicians reacted to this disease in practice at a time when it had become a fixture in early modern society. On the selection, one can document both the contributions of their study to the enrichment of our knowledge as well as the limitations of their utilization, which historians must take into account when studying consilia literature.

One of the most important limitations is the small numbers of the target groups of patients. Only the upper classes of society could afford consilia. Moreover, the authors of consilia, university-educated physicians, represented a minority within the entire range of established health-care practitioners up until the 20th century and thus the least important sector of medical care. Despite this, their practical activities, which by means of consilia document the extent of their mutual contacts and the level and capabilities of treatment of the elite classes of the population at that time, should not escape our attention. Using consilia for syphilis patients, it is possible to demonstrate how consilia can be useful for gaining an idea about the general discourse, learning details about the lives of graduated physicians and their (wealthy) patients and demonstrating the variability of this genre and the opportunity to obtain information useful for the enrichment of our knowledge concerning the history of medicine and related fields.

I will therefore attempt to interconnect two medical phenomena of the 16th century, consilia literature and the French disease. Somewhat paradoxically, attention will be primarily focused on the neglected and little-known phenomenon, while on the other hand, the phenomenon that has attracted attention since it first originated and has been relatively well studied will have a complementary role. Because of the low level of awareness about consilia works, it is essential to start with the clarification of the definition, main characteristics, and structure of consilia together with the delimitation of this genre with respect to related forms of literature. I will further mention the previous stages of development and expound upon the continuity of medieval consilia with those of the early modern period, which will be presented in an analysis of consilia collections and anthologies of fifteen selected physicians of the 16th century.

The consilia contained in these collections and anthologies form the basis of the study. They were written by physicians in the course of the 16th century and most were published during that period, but several of the cited titles only appeared after a lengthier period of time had passed. Their authors were representatives of famous faculties of medicine and the personal physicians of the members of ruling families. However, for the sake of comparison, several representatives of less renowned, yet not insignificant, municipal physicians were also included. Italian faculties of medicine and their representatives represented the pinnacle of 16th century European university medicine. Here, exactly where consilia literature originated in the Middle Ages and spread north across the Alps to the rest of Europe, it was unthinkable not to select at least a few famous names from among the ranks of their professors. The need to include representatives of German medicine in this probe does not require lengthy deliberation. Just like the "epistolae medicinales genre," consilia found fertile ground for its enthusiastic perception and extensive development in Central Europe. Representatives of French consilia literature were then also included because of the fact that only in France can we find universities that could compete with the Italian institutions with respect to their fame and attendance. It is just this comparison with Italian "rivals" that promises interesting findings.

On the basis of the probe into the consilia collections penned by 15 physicians, it is possible to obtain enough evidence for the definition of the main characteristics of this genre, its differentiation from other forms of expert literature, determination of possible nuances and differences from the approaches of the authors of medieval consilia. One chapter will also focus on specific aspects of the consilia-literature of the 17th-18th centuries. The information obtained will help to paint a picture of the practices of elite physicians, their mutual communication, and indirectly describe the world and sufferings of their patients.

Although consilia usually only provide very basic information about the patient, even the mapping of the usually mentioned social status of patients and sporadically mentioned names, especially regarding well-known figures from political history, can deliver interesting results.

With regards to physicians, it will be most interesting to study the way in which the experts involved communicate with one another, information regarding collaboration and on the contrary even any potential conflicts and discrepancies in treatment. A more detailed perspective about the collections and anthologies is provided by new findings concerning how they were compiled, the publication process itself and interventions of editors, while the study of other paratext materials, such as dedication letters, is also not without interesting discoveries. Individual subsections and an overall summary, which will compare the conclusions from the analyses of Italian, German and French consilia literature, will be dedicated to these and the other points.

The main topic of the second part of the book will be the consilia for patients suffering from the French disease written by physicians, whose collections and anthologies will be expounded upon in the first thematic part. This would not be possible without the concise placement of this disease into its historical context and at least a brief comment about its ontology, which significantly differs from the older understanding of the disease due to the influence of new methodological trends. Without a historical excursion into the history of humoral physiology and pathology, it would not be possible to understand a whole range of information and opinions that appear in the course of researching individual consilia for the treatment of the pox. It will certainly be demonstrated that the detailed study of 16th century consilia literature is enriching and interesting and that even consilia can reflect new trends and directions, the influence of new discoveries and ideas – simply everything that formed and influenced medical discourse. We certainly cannot claim that we know about all the aspects of the history of medicine of that period or even everything about the French disease.

Bibliography

Arrizabalaga, Ion. "Problematizing Retrospective Diagnosis in the History of Disease," *Asclepio* 54, no.1 (2002): 51-70.

Černý, Karel. *Mor 1480-1730. Epidemie v lékařských traktátech raného novověku*, [*The Plague 1480-1730. Epidemics in Early Modern Medical Treatises*]. Prague: Karolinum, 2014.

Eckart, Wolfgang U., and Robert Jütte. *Medizingeschichte. Eine Einführung.* Cologne: Böhlau Verlag, 2007.

Karenberg, Axel. "Retrospective Diagnosis: Use and Abuse in Medical Historiography," *Prague Medical Report* 110, no. 2 (2009): 140-45.

Kümmel, Werner F. "De Morbis Aulicis: on Diseases Found at Court." In *Medicine at the Courts of Europe, 1500-1837*, edited by Vivian Nutton, 15-48. London: Routledge, 1990.

Montanus, Ioannes Baptista. *Consultationum medicarum opus absolutissimum.* Basel: Petri, 1565.

Porter, Roy. *The Greatest Benefit to Mankind. A Medical History of Humanity from Antiquity to the Present.* London: Harper Collins Publishers, 1997.

Stolberg, Michael. *Gelehrte Medizin und ärztlicher Alltag in der Renaissance.* Oldenbourg: De Gruyter, 2021.

2 Consilia Literature from the Beginning

Abstract

This section is devoted to the creation and rise of consilia literature from its formation in the 13th century to its spread throughout Europe in the 15th century. The reader is introduced to the paradigm of a consilium, the three developmental stages and the names of the famous authors of that time. The main attention is paid to the consilia literature in the 16th century. Six important Italian physicians, seven German, and two French physicians were selected, whose biographic sketches and analysis of the specifics of their consilia collections enabled insight into typical characteristics of consilia literature. The most interesting aspects of consilia of the 17th century to the 18th century were outlined in the brief survey as well.

Keywords: consilia genre, development, 16th century representatives, Italy, Germany, France

2.1 Definition of the Genre and the Paradigm of an Ideal Consilium

Today, the Latin term "consilium" is exclusively connected with the original meaning of this Latin word, the metonymic designation of an institutional group of experts, which is supposed to arrive at a collective decision. However, one of the many additional meanings of this word designates the expert advice of a qualified and experienced individual, which from the standpoint of consilia literature is the more important meaning because it influenced the genesis of an entire literary genre and even gave it its name in the 14th century. As mentioned above, a consilium was the written advice of a physician, who was asked by a colleague for assistance in resolving a case. The description of the patient and development of the situation to date was also usually in writing so the counselor also had to rely on secondary information when making his diagnoses. He had to arrive at the approach to treatment on the basis of his own experience, trust in his

Divišová, Bohdana, *Medical Case Studies (Consilia medica) of the Early Modern Period.*
Taylor & Francis Group, 2022
doi: 10.5117/9789463723640_ch02

own erudition and faith in the effectiveness of the medical science of the time. At the beginning of his consilia, the physician designated the patient's physical constitution and symptoms and then continued with the diagnosis often even including a prognosis. In the concluding therapy section, he submitted his proposal for the manner of treatment, prescribed medicines and described the dietetic principles in detail. As will be mentioned later, a consilium could also be just a record of what had already been done, a record of an actual medical consultation, which brings the consilia closer to related genres like historiae, casus, and observationes, which will be analyzed below.

The most significant benefit and at the same time innovation of consilia literature at the time of its genesis was the fact that it was connected with real life. In contrast to treatises or commentaries to Avicenna and other old authorities, which were stuck in the captivity of theory, the authors of consilia faced real challenges and problems. Consilia capture the information and methods upon which all decisions of the physician regarding the treatment of the patient were based and reflect his everyday professional activities. The written record represents the fundamental divide in differentiating between a consilia-visit with consultation, during which someone was given advice regarding a particular problem, and a consilia-file, which became a part of a professional file, which however was also related to scientific theories. At the time of their greatest flowering, consilia were published in large numbers because they represented proof of the erudition, esteem and success of their authors, while for readers they were not only informative, but also a demonstration of the merit of the medical arts.[1]

Medieval and early modern consilia were and are thought of by historians rather in connection with related genres or in the enumeration of the works of individual physicians. Thus, the twenty-year-old work of Italian authors J. Agrimi and Ch. Crisciani, "Les consilia medicaux" still represents the foundational and singular work covering the period of the genesis and formation of consilia literature.[2] Despite the problems that stood (and stand) in the way of the complete explanation of all aspects of this topic, the authors succeeded in defining this independent literary genre, explaining its genesis and development within the framework of the economic and scientific contexts of the period, defining the form of a classic "ideal" consilia

1 For more detail see Keil, "Konsilium," 1370. Many of the other claims of this author, for example that consilia were an important intermediary between academics and laymen, do not fully reflect reality. From the time of its genesis, the consilium interconnected physicians.

2 Agrimi and Crisciani, *Les consilia.*

and characterizing its individual components.[3] They even included the exploration of the connection of this genre to Classical and Arabic medicine and examined related medieval forms of medical literature in their study. Their linguistic analyses of consilia and their written expression are also very beneficial. Even though their work is based exclusively on studies of Italian medieval and early modern collections, they succeeded in outlining models of the structures and types of different consilia applicable throughout the period of the existence of consilia literature.

According to the authors, the codified structure of an ideal consilium is comprised of three parts. In the first, the physician evaluated and examined the current state of the patient, while the second and third parts contained the physician's instructions.[4] A consilium usually excels at illustrating a case, which first requires a description of the patient and the characteristics of his problems. In an ideal consilium, which is however rarely found, we can learn the name, gender, age, social status and physical constitution of the patient, which was essential information for all subsequent decisions.[5] However, a typical consilium was rather more concerned with the disease than the patient. The described symptoms were furthermore placed into the context of a dietetic regimen, which the patient was supposed to follow, and finally came the prescription of medicines with the designated dosages of individual ingredients and "technical" procedures – bloodletting, "cleansing," bathing, burning, or fumigating.

These three parts of consilia correspond to two different sections. The first deals with the diagnosis and the second, which depends on the first, contains the regimen and pharmacological treatment. Each of these three parts, the casus (case), regimen or diet and medicinalia (medicines) – together termed the cura (treatment) – may be structured differently and of course in different degrees of detail. The greatest variation is found in the first part (casus), which defines the disease: list of symptoms, illnesses and indications that the physician links to the causes and the particular component of the complex (humoral constitution) of the patient.[6] The physician also had

3 The main problem remains the small number of modern publications and summary works regarding the consilia works of one specific author or one geographic area within a specified period.

4 For more detail see Agrimi and Crisciani, *Les consilia*, 88-9.

5 Physical constitution, temperamentum, part of humoral theory is based on the teaching concerning the constitution of the body from four main fluids (humores). More detail in chapter 4.1.

6 Causes, symptoms and disease represented independent units in current medical science and did not have to be related to one another. For more see Maclean, *Logic, Signs*, 261-265.

to designate a hierarchy and relationships among causes, single out the primary disease from the derived and secondary illnesses, and formulate the diagnosis, prognosis and finally the therapeutic plan.[7] The "casus" could be in the form of a simple one-sentence notification, or even a very detailed and lengthy discourse. It is precisely this part of consilia that could easily turn into a controversial treatise in the style of a scholastic dispute or a theoretical analysis resembling a treatise.

The structure of the second part, the regimina, is more stable than that of the first. Here, the physician prescribed the patient a lifestyle (diet) he was supposed to adopt, and which was related to "sex res non naturales."[8] This involved so-called "non-innate things," which included activities and processes related to the surrounding environment that are essential to maintaining human life and health: respiration (air), eating and drinking, defecation, sleep and being awake, physical exercise and mental processes. In the event of immoderate behavior, these became the main cause of a disease. In consilia, the order and importance of the each of the six non-innates varied. Some could be omitted, while others were addressed extensively. We even find consilia in which these six "things" are dealt with in a single sentence.

With respect to the structure, the pharmacological part usually comes last. It was common for authors to find their own form for the organization of this section, for example, according to the effects of the medicines, manner of use or ingredients. In the course of the development of consilia, this part underwent a significant transformation in the scope of the terminology used. Formulations varied greatly because they depended on the orientation of the author and needs of the individual treatment of the patient. However, in later times authors began to feel the need to modify this part and more general rules for their order and application were adopted. In later times, it of course also depended on the approaches of the editor and printer.[9]

This three-step structure became the basis for the classification of consilia types. Two[10] authors, Agrimi and Crisciani, consider the three-part

7 For more details concerning the foundations of diagnostic methods see ibid., 276-332; García-Ballester, "Galen as a Clinician," 1640-1642; Hankinson, "Philosophy of Nature," 217-25.

8 For more details see chapter 4.1. More in-depth about these six "things" e.g. García-Ballester, "On the Origin," 105-15.

9 Very detailed information regarding the genesis and expansion of prescriptions and their collections in the early modern period can be found in the monograph by historian A. Rankin. For more see Rankin, *Panaceia's Daughters*," 63-77.

10 For details see Agrimi and Crisciani, *Les consilia*, 27-38. As they mention, it would be possible to use numerous other criteria, e.g., according to inclusion in a collection, type of consultation of

composition to be the ideal paradigm despite the fact that it effectively represents only one type of consilium. Of course, multiple variants can be found not only in the different stages of consilia development, but even for a single author, which applies not only to medieval consilia. In addition to three-part consilia, another two are considered basic types: consilia reduced to the therapeutic part composed of the regimen and pharmacological prescriptions, and consilia limited only to the pharmacological part. These three variants are found among the works of all important authors in the course of all the centuries in which consilia literature was cultivated. However, it is often impossible to verify whether a consilium was written in a given form or later shortened through editorial modifications for the purpose of its inclusion in a collection or for printing.

2.2 Related Genres

The approximate definition above enables the differentiation of the consilium from other medical literary genres that are considerably similar in structure, character and scope and can also concern individual diseases and treatments. These include records concerning practical medicine and surgery, treatises, "exempla" (examples), "mirabilia" (remarkable cases, miraculous cures) and "practica" (analogous to the current medical "Vademecum").[11] However, the most significant and closely related, at times merging, medieval genres are considered "experimenta, experta (prescriptions of proven medicines), pseudoconsilia (non-real consilia without a specific recipient), expert opinions ("court" opinions), plague consilia and regimina.[12] Because of their popularity and plentiful representation even within later humanistic medical literature, the final two genres deserve a more in-depth characterization.

Anti-plague consilia, or advice on how to protect oneself against the plague, are among the non-real consilia without a specific recipient. The

one or multiple physicians, type of disease and even sociological aspects, to classify the various types of consilia.

11 For differentiation of the terms exemplum, experimentum and consilium see Crisciani, "Consilia, responsi, consulti," 259-79, 264; Crisciani, "Exempla in medicina," 89-108, 93-9. At the time that consilia literature originated and bloomed, it was supposedly not an exceptional trend to transform a consilium into a monograph or integrate monographs into consila. It was also common for an author to attach particular consilia to larger and more general treatises, which resulted in tractatus cum consiliis. It was not even exceptional for authors to call their real consilia a tractatus. For more Agrimi and Crisciani, *Les consilia*, 18-26.

12 The closest genre in the Early Modern Period is however "epistolae medicinales," for more see chapter 3.2. of this work.

most important part of these consilia was the "regimen preservativum," the lifestyle that protects against the plague. The plague afflicted all social classes, so the protective advice was addressed to everyone, often taking into consideration the wealth of the addressed social group. In the 15th century, when the consilium became established as a standard genre and the plague became an endemic disease, consilia, which were written for a different purpose, also contained a special section about the plague.[13] "Regimina sanitatis" was one of the "most interesting, most readable and liveliest types of medieval medical literature."[14] Its boom as an independent genre took place at the time that consilia literature developed from the 13th to the 15th centuries.[15] They differed from consilia primarily in that they did not concern a particular disease and focused on the right regimen for maintaining health and not treating a disease. They did not contain a diagnosis or symptoms and the prescriptions and advice provided were generally applicable. However, in the event of the outbreak of the disease, they lost their validity.[16]

An analysis of the relationship of consilia to regimen that originated during the 14th and 15th centuries uncovered that a large number of medieval consilia do not describe as the topic one disease, but the protection of health same as the regimen genre. The authors of collections at that time evidently considered these general protective consilia to be of greater importance and placed them at the beginning. In a large number of the studied consilia, physicians did not waste time with discussions of symptoms and diseases and instead immediately offered therapies. These consilia are presented as regimina despite the fact that they have a characteristic attribute of a consilium – they were written at the request of a particular patient afflicted by a specific disease.[17] However, even standard consilia contain a regimen, diet and treatment advice. This mingling and merging of genres,

13 In the period of the second half of the 14th century, authors Agrimi and Crisciani noted a gap or at least a decrease in the number of consilia and expressed the conjecture that this could have been a consequence of the enormous plague epidemic in the first half of the 14th century. For more see Agrimi and Crisciani, *Les consilia*, 38.

14 Říhová, "Regimen sanitatis," 13.

15 For the history of the development and specific aspects of this literature see e.g., Říhová, "Středověká pražská regimina," 39-43; Říhová, "Regimen sanitatis," 13-28; Říhová, *Dvorní lékař*, 95-8; or Riha, *Meister Alexanders Monatsregeln.*

16 For more detail see Agrimi and Crisciani, *Les consilia*, 22; Schipperges, "Regiment der Gesundheit," 1309-15.

17 For more detail see Vermeer, "Johann Lochners 'Reisekonsilia'," 145-96; Riha, *Wissenorganisation.* Especially helpful for the topics covered are chapters "Ärztliche Konsilien: Die Behandlung von Gicht und Pest," 79-99 and the following chapter "Prophylaxe: Regimen sanitatis," 100-17.

as demonstrated below, is not something uncommon even in later periods. This can be easily noticed even in the titles, where individual advice is designated as "consilium sive [or] regimen, or regimen sive [or] consilium."[18]

2.3 Collections and the Genesis of Consilia Literature

As we can see from previous analyses, in its function and epistemological quality the consilium was the result of a combination of many elements, which made it exceptionally suitable for compilation in collections. It was precisely through collections and anthologies that consilia became one of the most widespread types of medical literature in the medieval and early modern periods. The creation of collections then reciprocally contributed to the stabilization of their typical character.[19] Already in the first decades of the 15th century, authors of consilia adopted more scientific criteria for the logic and style of writing so that physicians' consilia could be grouped into collections or anthologies and become more like other educational texts. The most important of these "textbooks" were "practica", and the creators of consilia collections usually followed their topological and topographical scheme of ordering from head to toe ("a capite ad calcem").[20] The use of consilia and their collections for didactic purposes was one of the main reasons for their popularity and spread throughout Europe.

The ordering of consilia into structured works however also led to a major change regarding the "documentary" characteristics of consilia. Publishers started to adapt materials designated for publication to their intent, which affected the thoroughness of consilia. Most often personal information about the patient and time data were removed because the scientific order of doctrinal classification did not require any time determinations. Significant modifications of texts, such as the reduction or leaving out of individual parts, evidently occurred, but it is very difficult if not impossible to capture

18 Agrimi and Crisciani, *Les consilia*, 22.

19 For more see idem., 62-86. Here, beside the typology of consilia, the authors also outline the typologies of their anthologies and chart the directions, modalities and purpose according to which anthologies were constituted. The first anthology in the true sense of the word, a collectio-corpus of one author, was supposedly the anthology of Taddeo Alderotti, who was also the first to use this type of professional file to a great extent.

20 According to the authors, the model for this ordering was the 9th book of Rhazes Almansor, which was rediscovered at this time for the university public. For more see Agrimi and Crisciani, *Les consilia*, 69-73. The next most important was evidently Avicenna's Canon. For more see Siraisi, *Avicenna in Renaissance Italy*.

these major changes. These issues as well as the question of the impact that the invention of printing must have had on the spread and use of consilia literature have so far remain unexplored.

Since classical times, discussions between a physician and patient, or expert discussions concerning a case between several physicians, resulted in texts that captured special situations.[21] This fact proves that at a certain level of medical epistemology, the need appeared to summarize information about the patient and development of the illness in writing so that these could be put in relation to general theory or individual therapeutic prescriptions. At the same time, this is proof that these works were always connected with the professional activities of physicians, their communication and the exchange of information with colleagues. Clues to these treatises can be uncovered among some authors representing the Salerno School of Medicine. In this sense, these texts can be considered as the predecessors of medieval consilia, even though they did not become their direct source. Arab physicians, who were no less important for European medicine, created or translated treatises about clinical cases, but their works, with the exception of Rhazes, could not influence the medieval consilium in any significant way in comparison with those of Galen and Hippocrates.[22]

Nevertheless, Consilia medica or medicinalia, which since the time of their genesis at the end of the Middle Ages, developed into one of the most interesting forms of medical literature, was surprisingly primarily modelled after legal literature.[23] The new legal science is connected with the earliest stages of the genesis of the first universities and thus law had the opportunity to influence the development of universities to a much greater extent than could for example philosophy.[24] And it is evidently not a coincidence that the founder of the genre of medical consilia, Taddeo

21 Authors Agrimi and Crisciani mention that already in the Corpus hippocraticum one can find four types of expert texts of the kind discussed. In connection with files that dealt with practice and influenced the genesis of consilia literature, see Arrizabalaga et al., *Galen and Galenism*, 1646-51. From among clinical cases, only the treatise "Pro puero epileptico consilium" seems to have been written in the form of consilia. In its extensive scope and division into chapters, this text resembles a monographic and specialized treatise, but is written in the form of question and answer.

22 Agrimi and Crisciani, *Les consilia*, 12. From among the works of the late Arabian period, the most important one for consilia literature could only have spread at the beginning of the 16th century. For more on the topic see Siraisi, "Avicenna and the Teaching," 63-78.

23 For more see Keil, "Konsilium," 1370; Crisciani, "Consilia, responsi, consulti," 259-79.

24 Meuthen, *Kölner Universitäts Geschichte*, 8-9. However, the formation of consilia would be unthinkable without the new natural-philosophical thinking. Natural philosophy, which gained independence in meaning in the 13th and 14th centuries, had, as in many other fields, a clear influence here. For more see Baader, "Anatomie, Konsilienliteratur," 127-41.

Alderotti, taught medicine at the University of Bologna, where at the time the older and renowned faculty of law dominated. From the very beginning, the study of law brought to the forefront a new and for the development of universities existentially important aspect: the connection with practice.[25]

With regards to logic and epistemology, law and medicine showed very significant analogies and so a close relationship was born between the faculties of law and medicine. On the one hand, this connection inspired the genesis of medical advice "from afar" and the early adoption of consilia for teaching.[26] However, on the other hand, this caused a mutual rivalry between the two faculties, categories of teachers and representatives of these "lucrative arts," who held a lot of influence in both the urban and university environments.[27] However, it is quite certain here that a fact which L. Brockliss mentioned in connection with consultation literature of the 18th century but which also certainly applied in the formation of consilia and their beginnings, played an important role: "... the practice of consulting by letter was encouraged by the contemporary concept of status. ... who made their livings using their heads rather than their hands were more highly honoured."[28]

2.4 The Initial Stages of Development and Representatives

The physician, Taddeo Alderotti (Thadeus Florentinus, d.1313), who taught medicine in Bologna from 1260 to 1305, is considered by most historians to be the creator of real consilia and consilia literature.[29] An entire range of the typical characteristics of consilia, e.g., the addressee, "sex res non naturales,"

25 The introduction of scientific law into practice was caused by the growing complexity and differentiation of living conditions first in the urban environment of Italy and subsequently north of the Alps.

26 The study of consilia was common and at Montpellier their study was supposedly already mandatory from 1240. For more see Siraisi, *Medieval and Early Renaissance Medicine*, 73. For more about the use of consilia for teaching students see chap. "Medical Education," 48-77.

27 This rivalry initiated among other things written "expert" disputes, which considered questions such as whether medicine or law is more useful, which of these fields is "more scientific," or which has a greater tradition. In addition to a desire for greater influence at the university and the better financial situation of lawyers in cities, their arrogance and jealousy of physicians played a significant role. Academic arguments also continued in the following centuries in the form of treatises, which included crude insults and accusations from both sides. For more see Thorndike, "The Debate for Precedence," 185-90.

28 Brockliss, "Consultation by Letter," 79.

29 Agrimi and Crisciani, *Les consilia*, 39, 62-4. For the most detailed work on this physician see Siraisi, *Taddeo Alderotti*; and Siraisi, "Two Models of Medical Culture," 77-99. They are mentioned

diet and pharmacotherapy, already appear in his most important consilia. Besides Taddeo Alderotti, the most important authors of consilia of this period are Arnaldo de Villanova (d.1311) and Guglielmo Corvi (d.1326). Alderotti's influence was however absolutely fundamental because his students included a large number of important physicians, who further formed the genre of consilia and many continued their careers at various universities as professors: Bartolomeo da Varignano (d.1318), Mondino de'Luzzi (d.1327) and especially Gentile da Foligno (d.1348).[30] Among the ninety preserved consilia by Foligno, G. Baader considers the consilium on the plague, which became a model for a similar French treatise that then served as the model for all of Europe north of the Alps, to be the most valuable.[31] The death of Gentile da Foligno concludes the first stage defined as the beginning of the process at the end of which consilia was a clearly defined genre.

The second stage continued until the first half of the 15th century and is connected with the names of renowned physicians like William de Brescia, Jacobus de Regio, Guillaume Boucher (d.1400), Marsilius de Sancta Sophia (d.1403), Antonio Cermisone (d.1441) and Ugo Benzi (d.1439).[32] At this time, the definition of the epistemological structure of consilia and their consolidation in the form of a canonical medical work took place.[33]

The final stage of development, which according to Agrimi and Crisciani ends with the death of Bavier Baviera in the year 1480, involved the standardization of consilia and the clarification of its scientific character. According to the authors, Bartolomeo Montagnana (d.1452) and Giovanni Matteo de Ferrariis de Gradi (d.1472) are the most important creators of consilia at this stage.[34]

Consilia literature also enjoyed popularity in the following centuries, but its beginnings will be forever linked to the development of new currents of thought at North Italian universities, which from their genesis until the late modern period represented the most important and actually almost the only centers of learned medicine. The influence of faculties of medicine on the development and formation of anthologies of consilia, the involvement of

as creators of consilia literature by e.g., Thorndike, "'Consilia' and More Works," 8; or Baader, "Anatomie, Konsilienliteratur," 133.

30 For more see French, *Canonical Medicine*. Gentile's consilia however are only mentioned very marginally, ibid., 277-9.

31 Baader, "Anatomie, Konsilienliteratur," 135-7.

32 For the consilia of the last named see Lockwood, "A Medieval Consilium," 5-8.

33 Agrimi and Crisciani, *Les consilia*, 39; Thorndike, "'Consilia' and More Works," 8.

34 For more detailed biographies and information about the physicians mentioned see http://www.treccani.it/enciclopedia.

students on their spread and classification as well as the growing interest in this genre at universities between the end of the 14th century and first half of the 15th century were absolutely decisive.[35] In connection with this, it is necessary to above all emphasize the North Italian universities, which possessed a level of quality with which no others could compare. A special place is reserved in particular for two: "artium et medicinae" in Bologna, which was from the 13th to the 16th centuries the center of the study of anatomy and natural sciences, and then of course in Padua, which developed into the most influential school of medicine of the 16th century.[36] The genesis and development of these universities was influenced by more fortuitous historical, economic and cultural conditions, e.g. the tradition of the Salerno School from which the faculty of medicine in Bologna adopted among other things the integration of surgery into medicine.[37] Of great significance was the high standing of legal science and medicine and their orientation on practice, the different structure of these so-called "student" universities, and last but not least the strong presence of laymen among the masters and students. At these faculties, the increase of a completely new study material from translation schools started to make itself felt earlier and more positively than elsewhere.[38] All of this made the North Italian faculties the undisputed centers of medical education of the late Middle Ages, renowned not only for teaching autopsies of human corpses but also consilia literature.[39]

The situation at universities in other parts of Europe was however different. The difference in the religious and the social climate and economic situation of countries north of the Alps naturally had to have an influence on even the opportunity of the perception of consilia literature and their own production. The authors of "Les consilia" briefly mentioned the spread of the knowledge and acceptance of consilia literature beyond the borders of Italy, but concentrated their attention in particular on France since

35 For more see Agrimi and Crisciani, *Les consilia*, 104; Siraisi, *Medicine and the Italian Universities*, passim.

36 Due to its importance, the history of the faculty of medicine in Padua has been studied by many historians; to name a few of the many: Klestinec, "Medical Education in Padua," 193-220; Siraisi, *Medicine and the Italian Universities*, passim; Bylebyl, "The School of Padua," 335-70. The authors of *Les consilia* also devoted special attention to Padua because most of the consilia of Cermisone and Montagnana were edited at this faculty. For more see Agrimi and Crisciani, *Les consilia*, 69.

37 For more see Siraisi, *Medieval and Early Renaissance Medicine*, 153-86; Jones, "John of Arderne," 289-321.

38 Baader, "Medizinisches Reformdenken," 269.

39 For more about the development of teaching at these faculties see Siraisi, *Medieval and Early Renaissance Medicine*.

Paris and Montpellier were home to faculties of medicine, which with their renown, importance and attendance could practically equal the North Italian universities.[40] They however stated with surprise that in medieval France only a very small number of isolated consilia were produced and virtually nobody engaged in creating their collections. Due to the size of those institutions and the renowned physicians there, this fact is surprising and is usually explained primarily by the particularities of the institutional French cadre, which differed significantly from the Italian universities. A well-documented practice of consultations existed in France, but it purportedly remained on the level of oral statements, while written forms of physicians' work were dominated by prescriptions, commentaries of Arab authors, specialized monographs and practical manuals.[41]

As will be demonstrated, in particular German-speaking lands became the primary "carriers" and users of consilia literature during the period of transition between the Middle Ages and the Early Modern period. The question of spreading knowledge of consilia into Central and Western Europe (other than France) has not so far been paid sufficient attention by historians of medicine. The main problem remains the small number of modern publications and summary works regarding the consilia works of one particular author or a single geographic region in a firmly defined period. Since it is exceedingly difficult to analyze the development and state of any historical phenomenon without knowledge of its beginnings and the circumstances surrounding its genesis, the routes by which they spread and documentation of knowledge of consilia literature north of the Alps will be here at least indicated in several examples.

As already mentioned, in the Middle Ages, the undergraduate students and assistants of the Italian masters included large numbers of "ultramontani," students from various parts of Europe beyond the Alps. However, students from German-speaking lands, who initially most often sought out Bologna, the center of anatomy, clearly predominated. Padua, whose popularity could not be equaled even by the strongly attended faculties in Ferrara and Pavia, surpassed Bologna in the 16th century.[42] One can assume that upon their return home students spread the new "modern" trends in medicine with

40 For more see de Ridder-Symoens, "The Mobility of Medical Students," 47-89.

41 For example, the very successful Parisian via pragmatica, which originated and developed already in the 14th century, supposedly did not have any influence on the development of French medicine and thus even on the development of consilia linked to practice. For more see Jacquart, "Medical Practice in Paris," 186-210.

42 For more see Meuthen, *Kölner Universitäts Geschichte*, 17; de Ridder-Symoens, "The Mobility of Medical Students."

which they became acquainted in Italy. Because of a lack of any studies regarding this issue, we must make do with the randomly uncovered cases of individual persons and universities that indicate that the assumption concerning the spread of consilia by students is correct.

One example could be a central figure of German humanism, historian and physician Hartmann Schedel (d.1514), who as a student of medicine in Padua collected and publicized the consilia of Cermisone and Montagnana, provided notes and as a practical physician in Nuremberg, wrote some himself.[43] Further documentation of the knowledge of consilia in German regions is the donation of a student of medicine in Erfurt, Hermann Ymeker of Herford (d.1459), who bequeathed the faculty his private library containing among others a collection of consilia of the renowned Italian physician Bartholomeo Montagnana (d.1452). Moreover, a so-called "Padua school," established by a Padua graduate of medicine Conrad Eckard, existed in Erfurt. This school ended the influence of the universities in Vienna and Paris on the local study of medicine, which certainly must have also manifested itself in the adoption of new trends in literature oriented on practice.[44]

The existence of consilia at German universities is also confirmed by the library of the university in Heidelberg. In his study "Die medizinische Fakultät im 15. Jahrhundert," historian L. Schuba mentions that among the manuscripts preserved in this library there are about fifty codices with copies of medical texts containing consilia in addition to glosses and commentaries,.[45] The personal physician to three prince-electors, Heinrich Krauel von Münsingen (d.1476), who turned to the previously mentioned Padua professor Bartholomeo Montagnana with a request for a consilium for his patient, also practiced in Heidelberg.[46] Knowledge of consilia literature at this time is also confirmed at the University of Cologne on the Rhine to which professor of medicine Bernardus von Loen bequeathed his library in 1461. Among a range of commentaries and dietetic works, it also contained the consilia of renowned Italian physicians Gentile da Foligno, Marsiglia di Santa Sophia and Guglielmo de Varignana.[47] A similarly valuable donation was made in 1482 by a London practical physician, who donated eleven manuscripts that included a copy of the collections of Montagnana's consilia

43 Ibid., 65. About these consilia and figures, see especially 57; or Siraisi, "Avicenna and the Teaching," 73. For biography and works and his preserved consilia in detail see Fuchs, "Schedel, Hartmann."

44 Abe, *Die Erfurter medizinische Fakultät*, 177.

45 Schuba, "Die medizinische Fakultät," 162.

46 Ibid., 181.

47 Meuthen, "Kölner Universitäts Geschichte," 122.

to All Souls College Library in Oxford.[48] The University of Vienna also came under the influence of the medical faculty in Padua and its representatives accepted consilia literature.[49]

The consilia genre was even known at the University of Prague. "Contra pestilentiam consilium," an unaddressed, "non-real" consilium-treatise, which like many other European works appeared in connection with reoccurring plague epidemics, was found preserved among the works of professor of the faculty of medicine Christianus de Prachaticz (d.1439).[50] This documentation is isolated, even though some facts can be found among other Prague professors that could imply the production of consilia.[51] Due to the influence of further political-religious developments, the consilia genre did not develop in any way at the University of Prague.[52]

Most of the examples given of the presence of consilia in countries north of the Alps attest rather to the knowledge and spread of anthologies and consilia of Italian origin, than their local production. This is however an incomplete, randomly selected extract from a very broad and not yet comprehensively researched literature, which is probably still to a greater extent hidden in manuscripts. The problem of an exact determination of the spread of consilia literature in time and by region cannot be resolved without the existence of modern publications with commentaries, individual studies and subsequent summary works defined more specifically in time and place.

2.5 Consilium and Consultation Literature in Subsequent Centuries – Bibliography

The development of the consilia genre in the later stages of the early modern period has not yet received more systematic attention despite the fact that

48 Maclean, *Learning and the Market Place*, 91.

49 Uiblein, "Beziehungen der Wiener Medizin," 143-78.

50 This physician gained fame more from his astrological works. For more see Hlaváčková et al., *Biografický slovník*, 36-7; Stehlíková, *Od anděliky*, 11-20; Prachaticz, *De sanguinis minucione*. For more about the influence of the plague consilia of Gentile da Foligno see Baader, "Anatomie, Konsilienliteratur," 133.

51 E.g. Albík of Uničov (d.1426) completed degrees in medicine and law at the University of Padua and cited a certain unspecified Thadeo several times in his works. It is possible that he meant the founder of this genre, the already often mentioned professor, Taddeo Alderotti. For more about the life and works of this physician see Říhová, *Dvorní lékař*.

52 The Hussite Revolution at the beginning of the 15th century caused the financial collapse of the university and the closure of the three higher faculties, which were only restored in 1622. For more see Svobodný, "Lékařská fakulta," 183-202; or Hlaváčková and Svobodný, *Dějiny lékařství*, 51-4.

the consilium literature of the 16th and 17th centuries has not completely escaped the attention of historians (note for example the studies from M. Calabritto).[53] We can confirm the unflagging popularity of consilia and consultations by taking a look at bibliographies of the period compilations were sparked by a growing number of expert publications on medical and natural-scientific topics.[54] Information from four bibliographies suffices to provide a basic orientation concerning the number of consilia and consultations.

The first of the selected bibliographies was published it 1590. Its author was French physician Pascal Lecoq (Le Cocq; Paschalis Gallus).[55] In the section titled "Consiliorum medicorum scriptores..." Lecoq listed 21 names of physicians, who he determined to have authored consilia; however, these included nine representatives of consilia literature of the 15th century.[56] Up until the year of the publication of his "Bibliotheka," he recorded only 12 authors of consilia that originated in the 16th century. Only a year after the publication of Gallus' bibliography, another, authored by Strasbourg University Professor Israel Spach, was published. This physician knew more about older authors of consilia, but his knowledge and lists of "modern" authors correspond to those in Gallus' work.[57] Although printing houses were very willing to publish medical records, and information concerning new publications in the early modern period, because the medical records were of intensive communication, one cannot expect that Spach would have noted a significant shift.

So let's jump forward a longer period of time and take a look at another important bibliography, this time from the pen of German physician Johann Georg Schenck.[58] In his "Biblia iatrica," which was published 18 years after the work of Israel Spach, one can already find 45 authors of consilia or

53 Calabritto, "Curing Melancholia," 627-64; Calabritto, "Medicina practica," 63-83.

54 For more on bibliographies in the given period see Brodman, *The Development*, 31-2; Maclean, *Learning and the Market Place*, 62; or Černý, *Mor 1480-1730*, 17-8. Preserved catalogs with the offerings from pan-European book fairs, the most important of which in the discussed period was the fair in Frankfurt, offer additional opportunities to obtain the necessary information. For more see e.g., Maclean, *Logic, Signs*, 47-9.

55 Gallus, *Bibliotheca medica*. For more about the author and ordering system see Brodman, *The Development*, 18-20.

56 Ibid., 459; about physicians such as Antonio Cermisone, Hugo Senensis et al. Find more about them in chap. 2.4. of this work.

57 For more see Spachius, *Nomenclator*, 14-6.

58 In the work of E. Brodman this bibliography was probably classified by mistake among bibliographies from the 2nd half of the 17th century and close attention was paid neither to it, nor the author.

consilia collections.[59] However, among them again appear ten names of renowned experts, who had authored their consilia in the previous two centuries,[60] and if from the remaining authors we then exclude those who Schenck recorded as authoring only prophylactic and anti-plague consilia, we obtain a list of 28 names.[61] One can thus say that the amount of consilia literature increased. Nevertheless, this result does not entirely convincingly document the great popularity of the genre.

The clearest overview concerning authors of consilia literature of the 16th century can be found in a bibliography separated from Lecoq's work by almost half a century – in "De scriptis medicis" of Flemish physician Johann Antonides van der Linden.[62] At the time of its first publication in 1637, 98 names of consilia literature authors were already known to "the compiler of the most complete bibliography of medicine published up to his time."[63] In his work, Linden only included printed published collections and anthologies, while both Lecoq and Schenck cite significant numbers of manuscript collections and copies of individual consilia in their bibliographies.[64] Let's keep in mind that the impact of printed consilia is incomparable to that of manuscripts.

If we take a closer look, we find that only four authors connected with the 15th century (Cermisone, Benzi, Baviero, da Foligno) appear in Linden's work; an absolute majority of the consilia and their collections – even those with publication dates at the start of the 17th century – are from the 16th century. Without the aforementioned medieval authors and those authors whose consilia collections cannot be found (Quercetanus, Stojus), we arrive

59 Schenckius, *Biblia iatrica.*

60 Hugo Senensis, Gentile da Foligno, Bartholomeo Montagnana, Antonio Cermisone, Thaddeus Florentinus (Alderotti) and others appear again. However also "captured" are the consilia of German physician Hartmann Schedel. Schenckius, *Biblia iatrica*, 215.

61 Unreal and prophylactic-focused consilia were not included in this list.

62 Johann Antonides van der Linden (1609-1664), for more see Brodman, *The Development*, 29-36.

63 Ioannes Antonides Lindenius, *De scriptis medicis*, 532-5. The consilia was included in the second book in the section "Medicina Specialis."

64 A telling example for all others is German physician Antonius Niger, about whom Schenck mentioned: "Eiusdem consilia M.S. servantur apud Casparum Schwenckfeldt medicum" [His manuscript consilia are kept by physician K. Schwenckfeldt]. Schenckius, *Biblia iatrica*, 64. A similar reproachful note can be found by the name of the renowned J. Guinther von Andernach, where Schenck directly reproaches his colleagues for guarding consilia like dogs and not providing them to the public to the detriment of future generations. "...in varios morbos consilia dedit, latent hactenus apud nonnullos, qui non aliter atque canes ..., defraudata omni posteritate, advigilantes servant." Ibid, 311. It should be noted that the impact of printed consilia is not to be compared with that of manuscripts.

at only 31 names of consilia authors. Most publications are not collections of consilia of a single author, but anthologies comprised of the consilia of dozens of experts.[65] However, in his bibliography, Linden treated consultations as an independent genre and separated observations, or letters (epistolae), which for example Pascal Lecoq either didn't register at all, or added to the list of consilia.[66] If we were to also add the collections of related genres to the authors of consilia, the list would also include 19 names of consultation authors, 110 authors of medical letters and responses,[67] and 19 physicians who recorded medical observations.[68] These facts are already more comforting and the strict division of these genres moreover bears witness to the evident consolidation of the epistemological boundaries between closely related genres. These boundaries were however created artificially, so it is not surprising that they manifest as very fluid in literary practice.

Physicians from German lands, or countries counted among those speaking German (Austrian lands, Switzerland, today's Netherlands and Belgium, Denmark) predominate among the authors of consilia and other closely related genres in Linden's bibliography.[69] The second most numerous group is comprised of Italian physicians, while authors of other nationalities (France, England, Spain) have minimal representation. However, the above-mentioned facts cannot be considered as absolutely authoritative. Firstly, these are exclusively printed published collections and we do not know how many consilia failed to find a publisher, many collections were published long after the author's death and the possibilities of the authors of bibliographies to gather information were limited by the times, so Linden's list most certainly does not correspond to reality.

The final bibliography that we will take a look at is the so-called "Lindenius Renovatus" first published in the year 1686. It was based on Linden's

65 Four extensive anthologies compiled by Lorenz Scholz (1598), Joseph Lautenbach (1605), Iohannes Wittich (1606) and Johannes Phillip Brendel (1615) are the most important works for consilia of the 16th century.

66 Schenck verifiably planned to create special bibliographies divided by the nationality of the author, or according to his orientation towards for example alchemists, paracelsians, etc.; but this plan was evidently never realized.

67 Lindenius, *De scriptis*, 478-9. Ibid. on the page 480 "Responsa" (answers) are presented in a separate section. Their authors – except for one – are mentioned in the same work among the authors of consultations.

68 For more on the formation of distinct medical genres in the 16th century see Pomata, "Praxis Historialis," 105-46.

69 However, if this first impression is confirmed, it would interestingly correspond with the findings that N. Siraisi expressed concerning the publication and popularity of epistolic literature in the same century. For more see Siraisi, *Communities of Learned Experience*.

aforementioned bibliography which German physician Georg A. Mercklin expanded with new additions and authors.[70] The amount of medical literature was already so great that it was necessary to publish the indices in a separate volume called the "Cynosura."[71] Mercklin's approach to ordering and naming individual genres was simplified compared to Linden's. After searching the term "Consultationes," the reader is referred to "Consilia;"[72] medical correspondence was left a separate section, other closely related genres (e.g., "Casus") were categorized with the observations.[73] At the end of the 17th century, G. A. Merclin knew of 105 physicians who wrote consilia or consultations. He mentioned 97 authors of observations, but only named 52 physicians from among the letter writers.[74] Naturally, this information needs to be taken with a considerable grain of salt; all authors of the named genres of the 16th and 17th centuries are most certainly not captured, while on the other hand, classical and medieval authorities are mentioned.

Even much newer and more reliable sources corroborate the unflagging interest in this type of consultation among physicians and publishers. The creators of a digital project that focused on the collection, documentation, categorization and research of medical correspondence in the early modern period also included consilia in the subject of their study.[75] Although the project focuses on the correspondence of physicians from historically German lands, more than 500 consilia and consultations have been discovered so far and almost 200 of their authors have been identified by name. If we consider that only part of the European community of that time is in the "crosshairs," and the results cannot yet be definitive, it is clear that adding up the preserved consilia and consultations from all over Europe would give us a very large number.

We are informed (however concisely and incompletely) about the extent of the popularity of consilia literature among physicians and their patients. However, we know nothing for example concerning the writing styles of the individual consilia of specific physicians, the process of working consilia into collections, about editorial work and the range of other information that consilia can provide. In order to obtain a perfect overview of the consilia works of this period, it would of course be necessary to submit individual

70 Mercklinus, *Lindenius Renovatus.*

71 Mercklinus, *Cynosura medica.*

72 Ibid., 36. "Consultationes: Vid. Consilia Medica."

73 Ibid., 44-5 "Epistolae Medicae;" 27 "Casus Medicinales: Vid. Observationes Medicae."

74 Ibid., 99-100 "Observationes Medicae;" 44-5 "Epistolae Medicae."

75 Frühneuzeitliche Ärztebriefe des deutschsprachigen Raums (1500-1700), www.aerztebriefe.de [12.1.2021]

consilia to analysis, process the individual collections of consilia from different authors, compare differences and similarities, and do so if possible, from the origination of this genre up to the 17th century. In the course of this process, it would be appropriate to take into account the language of the physician, his "confessions" both religious and professional (Galenism – Paracelsianism) and whether these facts were reflected in the approach to the rendition of consilia, treatment or patients. Additionally, the period in which the consilia originated, publication years of collections, dates and modifications in republications, consideration of epistemological quality, quantity and additional aspects should not be left aside.

From this list of requirements, it is evident that they cannot be fully realized, at least not now and by one researcher. Consilia literature does however deserve attention. For this reason, some of the tasks mentioned above will be selected and using these we will try to expound the motivations of individual participants of the consilium process, show possible similarities of consilia, approaches and reasons for the publications of consilia collections, and to obtain interesting information in order to enrich the history of medicine. This attempt to answer certain questions concerning consilia production will be limited to the 16th century, while consilia and collections created up to the end of the 17th century will occasionally serve as comparative materials. The purpose of this overview is to outline the possibilities and potential direction of future research.

2.6 Selected Representatives of Consilia Literature of the 16th Century

There is a relatively small number of studies devoted to consilia, consultations and their authors in the 16th century, so a more concise handling and treatment of the topic is not possible. In order to examine the epistemological development and specific characteristics of consilia literature in this period, one can utilize time-delimited probes that focus on only several physicians and the fates of their consilia. Although such a study will be selective and only indicative, it could at least draw attention to some interesting facts and differences among different collections and authors. 15 representatives of the medical community and consilia literature from Italy, France and the German lands will be at the center of our attention. These figures have been selected in order to represent all decades of the 16th century, but slight overlaps with the previous and subsequent centuries are unavoidable. The list of the names of the selected physicians is in the order of their dates of birth. Brief biographies with an analysis of their consilia collections, which are the topic of the following chapter, are only partly ordered by dates, while the primary basis was the language (or nationality) of the physicians.

Benedetto Vettori (1481-1561)
Giovanni Battista da Monte (1489-1551)
Vittore Trincavelli (1496-1568)
Jean Francois Fernel (1497-1558)
Antonius Maria Venusti (turn of the 15th and 16th cent.-1570s)
Johann Crato von Krafftheim (1519-1585)
Girolamo Capivaccio (beg. 16th cent. -1589)
Reiner Solenander (1524-1601)
Cristoforo Guarinoni (1534-1604)
Diomedes Cornarius (1535- approx. 1599)
Johann Wittich (1537-1596)
Guillaume de Baillou (1538-1616)
Lorenz Scholz (1552-1599)
Thomas Mermann (1559-1622)
Johannes Matthaeus (sec. half of the 16th cent.-first half of the 17th cent.)

The selection of the figures listed above was not limited to representatives of one school or one specialization. The common denominator among these physicians was their knowledge, success and renown, thanks to which they were asked by colleagues for advice. The reach and extent of their professional influence in their eras varied and do not necessarily fully correspond with the scope of our contemporary knowledge of their life fortunes and works. Representatives of the physician-counsellors include members from the different levels of the hierarchy of this profession, including those representing physicians in different "forms of employment" – from simple municipal doctors (Venusti, Scholz) to professors at important universities (Vettori, da Monte, Trincavelli, Fernel, Capivaccio, de Baillou) to even the personal physicians of crowned heads (Crato, Solenander, Guarinoni, Cornarius, Wittich, Mermann, Matthaeus). Of course, the careers of many physicians unfolded in steps and thus they could have held all the aforementioned positions. Some even held these posts concurrently (e.g. Fernel, de Baillou).

When researching the collections of these figures, particular attention was paid to the circumstances that preceded or accompanied the creation of collections or anthologies, in addition to the persons to whom the works were dedicated and the reasons for this, and finally to the motives behind the writing or compiling of collections. The figure of the editor, who represents an important factor, attracts no less attention. It could be quite important whether the editor was the author himself, or it is necessary to account for the interventions of other persons who influenced the order of the consilia, their structure, the number of mentioned details or dating. An important question is even the number of consilia published in different collections or anthologies. The most important authors of the end of the 15th century account for hundreds of consilia, and as long as the popularity of consilia literature was increasing, it could have been reflected in the numbers of consultations in one volume. The difficult to answer question of whether the published consilia were actual "remote" advice sent in the form of a letter, or rather supplementary records, deserves greater attention. Observations concerning these details could set another direction for research concerning both consilia as a genre as well as related categories (observatio, epistolae etc.).

As we know, information concerning patients does not tend to be extensive at all, so the center of attention will be exclusively on information about their social standing (if mentioned) and random pieces of interesting information like the names of famous families or figures, or as the case may be, the representation of patients of various nationalities among individual physicians. Although this "screening" is quite superficial, it could provide information that could shed an interesting light even on the personality of a physician, the everyday routine of his profession and of course the possible relationship with the patient or his attending physician, collaboration among physicians themselves or professional institutions. They may also however be significant for the explanation of certain areas of the epistemology of consilia literature, or even touch upon "great" political history. The names of the presented diseases and symptoms and their treatment, or if pertinent the division of consilia into groups according to the disease have been left aside because this issue would require a separate study for each of the consilia collections. The exception however will be consilia regarding the "French disease" which will be covered in a separate chapter.

2.7 Representatives of Consilia Literature in 16th Century Italy

The earliest among the researched physicians was evidently Benedetto Vettori (Benedictus Victorius, 1481-1561), who was born in the northern Italian city of Faenza. After his studies at the Faculty of Medicine of Bologna, he successfully practised medicine in various Italian cities. In 1534, he became a professor of medicine in Padua, and six years later he accepted a professorship at his "alma mater" in Bologna, where he then taught until his death.[76] He was considered one of the best philologists of his day and is the author of a range of comprehensive commentaries to Hippocrates and practical medical works, including one of the first works about the French disease. His collection, the "Medicinalia consilia" was first published in 1551 in Venice at the expense of printer Vincenzo Valgrisi, who dedicated this book to the renowned physician and botanist Pietro Andrea Mattioli (1501-1577) as thanks for his recovery.[77] The same dedication is found in the second edition published five years later, which I am using because it was expanded by the publisher to include newly written consilia.[78] In the preface, Vettori presents the reason for the publication of his consilia (according to Galen's example) as being that they "... explain the different constitutions of various people, their diseases and locations."[79]

Vettori's collection includes 44 consilia that are quite extensive because this physician placed great emphasis on a detailed regimen for the patient. He devoted a separate paragraph to each of the so-called "sex res non innates." Special attention is devoted to foods, which were divided in detail into types (fish, meat, vegetables, cheeses, wine etc.). Dates, location of the composition of consilia and names of patients do not appear with any regularity. However, the social status of patients is commonly given, which confirms that the addressees of consilia tended to have higher social status. For example, a range of consilia so described by Vittori were intended for the Bishop of Trento. Interesting is the first consilium, which confirms that consilia could only be a written record of an actual consultation of several physicians and that it evidently was not uncommon to address a request for medical advice simply to a faculty instead of a particular physician.[80]

The next three physicians were also professors, but this time from the Padua Faculty of Medicine. Their teaching and work influenced more than one generation of physicians throughout Europe, which was the reason for their selection for this study. The first and evidently most important of them is

76 Hirsch, *Biographisches Lexikon*, 102. Surprisingly, the name of this author is not included in modern Italian biographies.

77 Victorius, *Medicinalia consilia,* 1551. In consilia at the beginning he thanks Mattioli even for entrusting his workshop with the publication of the commentaries to Dioskorides. Ibid., 2r.

78 Victorius, *Medicinalia consilia,* 1556.

79 Ibid., a 4r. "... diversas hominum naturas explicant et varias eorum affectiones, atque loca."

80 Ibid., 22v. "Initum est consilium [took place] in Patavino gymnasio 1535. 24.9., et ex omnium doctorum consensu a Benedicto Victorio Faventino editum. [and with the consent of all was written by B. Victorius]."

Giovanni Battista da Monte (Ioannes Montanus, 1489-1551), who was born into a noble family in Verona and completed his studies of medicine in Padua.[81] After several years of practice in Brescia, he undertook a journey around various Italian cities and worked on translations of classical medical works.[82] In 1542, he was offered a professorship of practical medicine at the University of Padua, which he of course accepted. He was one of the first professors who regularly visited Padua hospitals with his students during practical instruction and is thus often considered the founder of clinical instruction. His work influenced many students from virtually all countries in Europe. His translations were already widely published during da Monte's lifetime; however, his expert medical works were published posthumously thanks to his devoted students, which also applies to the collection of his consilia. Their most complete edition was the work of the no less renowned physician Johannes Crato of Krafftheim in the year 1565.[83] The first volume is comprised of common consilia, mostly discussing the illness of a patient, who da Monte did not see and about whose condition he was informed by letter. The second volume, edited by Crato, however includes detailed reconstructions of cases based on direct observation.[84]

In the dedication to the Senators of Wroclaw, we can read of the reasons that moved Crato to publish a comprehensive edition of da Monte's consilia: firstly, it was an effort to "somehow help human society ...;"[85] another was of course to express respect to a beloved professor and his knowledge and last but not least, to provide a clear methodological instruction and summary of the right foundations of medicine for young physicians and students, whom Montanus's works were to protect from "pernicious ideas."[86] Crato did not neglect to thank his fellow students, who contributed with their records of da

81 Di Mucillo, "Da Monte, Giovanni."

82 Starting in 1533, he served for a short time as the personal physician of Cardinal Ippolito de´ Medici.

83 Montanus, *Consultationum medicarum opus*. The name of the work, which mixes the terms "consultation" and "consilium," documents the identical meaning of these terms.

84 In this volume Crato also included the treatment of fevers, which are also detailed descriptions of directly observed cases and contain instructions on how to write a consilia related type of "historiae." This fact, just like additional details regarding other practical works by da Monte, was pointed out by historian G. Pomata, who here sees a significant shift in the epistemological level. For more see Pomata, "Praxis Historialis," 128-9.

85 Montanus, *Consultationum medicarum opus*, 2r. "aliquid communi hominum societati adiumenti conferre..."

86 Ibid. This was probably an allusion to Paracelcism in general, which Crato hated, but could also have referred to the ongoing professional dispute between physician Giovanni Argenterio (d. 1572) and Giulio Alessandrini (Iulius Alexandrinus, d. 1590), who was Crato's friend and colleague in imperial service. For more see Siraisi, "Giovanni Argenterio," 328-55.

Monte's consilia, which "with great effort and care, he corrected, added missing parts and removed distorted parts ..."[87] This is confirmation of the selectiveness of an editor when working with consilia, but it is clear that Crato (like other editors) showed himself to be conscientious because each time he noted his changes to the text.[88] In consilia captured by students while accompanying their professors around hospitals, even dates, locations and especially the opinions-consilia of other physicians who were in the advisory collegium, were recorded. Crato even mentioned his work on da Monte's consilia in one of the letters to his friend, the Nuremburg physician Joachim Camerarius, with words that must bring a smile to the face of anyone who has ever edited anything: "Correcting consultations makes my blood boil to the point that I can hardly keep myself from stomping on the book, but I will persevere."[89]

A total of 434 consilia divided into two parts were included in the entire collection. The first part contained 384 consilia classified according to the type of disease into coherent groups, while the second part with 50 consilia was devoted solely to fevers.[90] Names of patients are not uncommon, but in a large number of consilia, those specified by the name of the patient are nonetheless in the minority. Dates are more common and confirm that the consilia are mainly from the time da Monte spent at the university. Among the other collections, da Monte's is truly exceptional because it includes a large number of records of actual consultations with colleagues, which is evidenced by the initial address or even name of the consilium.[91] Perhaps precisely for this reason, many of them were originally in Italian.[92]

Da Monte's patients included representatives of Italian patrician families as well as representatives of the nobility from across Europe, including those from the German lands, Poland, Hungary and Spain.[93] A peculiarity

87 Montanus, *Consultationum medicarum opus*, 3v. "... singulari studio et diligentia emendavi, quaeque deesse videbantur, adiunxi: quae depravate accesserant, sustuli, ..."

88 Ibid., e.g., Cons. XLVIII., 126. "Hoc in loco poteram aliquid monere de correctione..." [Here I could mention something about the correction].

89 Crato, *Consiliorum liber quintus,* 313. "Emendatio consultationum saepe ita mihi movet stomachum, ut vix me continere possim, quin interim librum pedibus teram, sed emendabo tamen."

90 To the system of compiling this work see Calabritto, "Curing Melancholia," 632-3.

91 Montanus, *Consultationum medicarum opus,* 1. Cons. I., De ophiasi ... dicta in colloquio cum chirurgo et D. Frisimelico. Anno 1547, 16. 3.

92 Ibid., e.g., 59, Cons. XXIIII.; 184, Cons. LXXV.

93 Ibid., e.g., 72, Cons. XXXI. ... pro Ill. Matrona a Ditrichstain Germana; 138, Cons. LIII. ... pro Ill. Duce Bavariae. Datum anno 1546; 270. Cons. CXI. ... pro ... Germano Fuggero datum 1548; pg. 273, Cons. CXII. Ill. D. Aloisio Gonzagae; 321, Cons. CXXXI. ... pro ... ducissa Urbini; 362, Cons. CL. ... pro gen. D. Adamo a Dietrichstein, Anno 1546, etc.

of da Monte's consilia remains that because of his visits to hospitals, even members of the lower social classes and thus children of these classes appear in his collection, which is not at all common among other authors.[94] Even (for us) amusing anecdotes, which uncover the human side of da Monte's approach to patients and document the daily realities of physicians, can be found among the descriptions of cases. In the introductory commentary to one of the consilia on which he collaborated with a colleague, we can read:

> "… After a discussion, Frisimelica prescribed a manner of diet, which Montanus concluded must be modified so that they would not have to listen to such complaints as are made about the physicians of Cracow. Patients complained that these physicians almost tortured them to death with a strict diet. Then, Montanus proposed this consilium, which follows."[95]

Montanus's successor at the University of Padua was Vittore Trincavelli (Victorius Trincavellius, 1496-1568), who studied medicine at the universities in Bologna and Padua, where he graduated. After graduation he returned home to Venice, where he soon gained renown through his selflessness during an outbreak of a plague epidemic on the island of Murano. In 1551, he assumed the chair of professor in Padua after his above-named colleague and worked there until 1568, when he left to work as a physician in Carinthia. However, in this same year he returned to his hometown and died shortly thereafter. His educational work influenced many students and as a representative of a philologically oriented generation of professors, he promoted the publication of old classics, but at the same time was also among the most respected practical physicians.[96]

Trincavelli's collection of consilia was only first published 18 years after his death.[97] Its editor was the author's son Bernard, who in the dedication of the work to the Padua prosecutor mentioned that after the Europe-wide success of his father's philosophical and medical works, he had decided to also publish the rest of the documents in his possession, his father's consilia and letters.[98] The subsequently printed eulogy noted the fame of this physician

94 Ibid., 98, Cons. XXXIX. Pro puero hebraeo epileptico … recitante doctore casum; 885, Cons. CCCLXX. Pro puero in hospitali; 887, Cons. CCCLXXIII. De scate pro puero, dicta in hospitali.; 628, Cons. CCLXII. De hydrope pro puero in hospitali S. Francisci.

95 Ibid., 150, Cons. LIX.

96 For more di Fortuna, "Trincavelli, Vittore."

97 Trincavellius, *Consiliorum … libri tres.*

98 Ibid., 2r.-2v. "…cum intelligerem alia quoque illius opera, quae apud me extant adhuc, expectari quam avidissime, ut ego hoc tempore statuerim Epistolas et Consilia medica in lucem proferre."

even in mentioning that his patients were from throughout Europe.[99] In this collection, a total of 91 consilia were published in three books. Individual consilia are detailed, but unfortunately the name of the patient or the date was not recorded very often. The few dated consilia were written in the 1550s and 1560s. The formal introductory remarks indicate that these consilia were often for a patient who was not seen and his attending physician, and also unsurprisingly that the person was wealthy and distinguished.[100] It is remarkable that in at least one consilium Trincavelli expressed a concern about the correctness of his diagnosis and the need to see the patient.[101] His concern was not isolated, as evidenced by physician Laurenz Scholz (see below). Trincavelli's collection surprisingly ends with the 87th consilium. The following "consilia" are actually medical treatises.[102] It is not possible to determine why these treatises were designated as consilia and why they were not published separately.

There was evidently interest in Trincavelli's works because his collection of consilia was published again a short time later in Lyon and especially in Basel by Johannes Waldkircher, one of the most important European printers, who specialized in the publication of medical literature.[103] Although only a year passed between the Venetian and Basel editions, the rendition in the ordering and adaptation of the consilia is quite different. A comparison of the approach of the new editor may serve as minor documentation of the epistemological development of the genre. Johannes Waldkircher provided not only the publication, but also the preface and dedication, which he devoted to the renowned Danish physician Petrus Severinus. In addition to a glowing recommendation of the services of his friend, a Danish bookseller (which was probably the reason for the dedication), many remarkably interesting things appear in the subsequent preface. In addition to discussing interesting points from history, for example, concerning the Alexandrian

99 Ibid., 5v. "Qui quaeso hac aetate insigni aliquo malo aegrotarunt aut Italiae duces, aut Germaniae, seu Galiae vel Hispaniae princeps fuerint, qui non huius vel opem, vel consilium, vel praesentiam cupide quaererent et implorarent?"

100 Ibid., 4r. Cons. IIII. Pro Consiliario ... Regis Romanorum...; 82r. Cons. LXII. Pro Marchione quodam... ; 57v. Cons. L. Pro Cardinali laborante tussi ... etc.

101 Ibid., 61v. Cons. LII. "... mihi tamen adhuc admodum videtur difficile iudicium de illis resolutum affere: praesertim cum absens sim, necque ullam alioquin cognitionem possim mihi comparare inspiciendo et oculis observatione ..." [It seems too hard for me to decide when I'm not present ... and I can't compare it to my own observation...]

102 Ibid., 111v. Cons. LXXXVIII. Sermo de cordis affectibus.; 112v. Cons. LXXXIX. Sermo de animi defectu.

103 Trincavellius, *Consilia medica* 1587. For more about important publishing houses see Maclean, *Learning and the Market Place*, 62.

school, astronomy and the history of the University of Padua, he even noted new diseases including the French disease.[104] He also mentioned the manner of the acquisition of new consilia and the reason for the new organization of the collection:

> "Since the public benefit and with even the aid of results, the consilia and letters of professor of medicine V. Trincavelli were published in the past two years according to the example of [Montanus], first in Venice and then in Lyon, but everywhere in the same spirit. Because many of the consilia of this author were in private hands of those, who he taught and advised, these people gladly provided them for the general welfare, to contribute to the sacred treasury of medicine and so that they could all be published together. Among those who helped the most are the renowned German physicians: Kielmann, Camerarius, Fritsch, Zwinger and Schenck. However, the consilia are of three types: those written and sent, those presented as lectures in schools (only a small number of these) and those pronounced at consultations (which are generally called collegia). This was the reason why the consilia of others were added. Because T[rincavellius] received the initial statements to the final opinions and conclusions, it is necessary to evaluate all of his views in comparison with the opinions of others in order to recognize what T[rincavellius] considered right in medicine, what to allow and what to reject. For this reason, it was essential to add the consilia of others here. Furthermore, this edition is special in particular because ... it is organized according to bodily cavities: previous editions lacked this clear order. Finally ... that, which was not of great benefit for medicine other than for persons and certain circumstances, was removed."[105]

Firstly, here the publisher confirmed that German students contributed quite significantly to the spread and growth of consilia literature. Furthermore, as the editor, he considered it important to explain the existence of the names of other physicians in a collection published under the name of Trincavelli and used the types of consilia for explanation, which evidences the unambiguity of the epistemological view of the genre. Furthermore, as he emphasized, everything unnecessary for treatment was removed, the result of which all the personal formulations of physicians, which show the relationship to the patient or attending physician, disappeared. Because

104 Trincavellius, *Consilia medica*, 3v.
105 Ibid., 4r.-4v.

of this decapitation of the consilia, we cannot determine whether those consilia published by Bernardo Trincavelli were included in Waldkircher's collections. The loss of specific information about patients, as well as all other editorial changes, the division of consilia into groups according to the diseases of different parts of the body make consilia collection more like collections of "practica" and attest to an effort to give the consilia collection a more universal applicability and imprint it with a more scientific character according to the dogmatic methods of the time.[106]

As already stated, the collection is divided into three books according to the most important bodily cavities. The first book "De morbis capitis et partium eius" (Concerning Diseases of the Head and its Parts) contains a total of 76 consilia, the second "De morbis thoracis" (Concerning Diseases of the Chest) includes only 16 consilia, while the third "De morbis infimi ventris" (Concerning Diseases of the Lowest Cavity), which is divided into other individual "cavities" or organs, (e.g., De affectibus ventriculi), is comprised of 127 consilia. In total, the collection contains 249 consilia, but as reported by the editor in the preface, most were contributed to by another three or four physicians through the expressions of their opinions. The most frequent consultants usually included other professors of the Padua faculty Gabriele Falloppio, Luigi Bellocato, Basiano Landi, Antonio Fracanzani and Francesco Frigimelica. For each case, several consilia-advices were prepared remotely, or physicians were present at the patient's side, forming an actual contemporary consilium, and then only recorded their opinions in writing. Perhaps this is a similar situation to that of da Monte's consilia: the physicians involved only expressed their opinions orally and students captured them in writing. If all the consilia in the collection are then included, the actual number nears at least 700. The inclusion of the consilia of all participating physicians is important not only for the reasons mentioned in the preface by Waldkircher. For us, even for example the information that one of the most important anatomists of the time, Gabriele Falloppio, could be viewed as a creator of consilia, even though neither Lecocq nor Linden mention him in their lists of consilia authors at all, is beneficial. It is of course a question whether it is at all possible to include him and the other mentioned physicians among the authors of consilia, if we do not know whether they wrote their own consilia, or even whether they would agree to the inclusion of their advices and their printed publication under the summary designation of "Trincavelli's Consilia."

106 For more see Wear, "Explorations in Renaissance Writings," 125-6.

The last of the representatives of the Paduan professor staff presented here is Girolamo Capivaccio (Hieronymus Capivaccius, 1523-1589), who was a generation younger. He was from an important noble family from Padua and completed his studies of medicine in his home town. He started teaching at his alma mater in 1553 as a "professor extraordinarius."[107] In 1564 he became a regular professor of practical medicine and essentially held this position until his death. In 1576, together with his colleague and rival, the today much more famous Girolamo Mercuriale, he became an evaluator of a contagion that broke out in Venice. Their "consilium" ended in a fiasco, which negatively impacted the reputations of both physicians.[108] Despite this, Capivaccio remained a sought-after expert, especially for the treatment of fevers and syphilis. He died in Mantua while treating the local duke.

His consilia were published in the comprehensive work "Opera omnia," which saw the light of day after the death of its author. The publication was arranged by his former student, the Frankfurt physician Johann Hartmann Beyer and the work was dedicated to the Archbishop of Mainz.[109] The expansive and flowery reason elaborated for the publication of the works of the Paduan professor did not present anything unusual: respect for the teacher, an effort to preserve his fame and an example for subsequent generations, emphasizing the great significance of medicine for the life of a person. However, it interestingly comments on the need for a new edition of the practical part, which according to all accounts was only published eight years before: the need to cleanse it of the "foulness" of French and Italian typographers.[110] Capivaccio's consilia were placed in the fourth part, called the "Mista" (mixta) and it seems that these consilia were obtained by the editor during his studies in Padua. In total, only 51 consilia are presented, but Capivaccio was not the sole author of all of these by far. In some cases, either several participants are signed under one consilium, or each physician expressed his opinion on one patient in his independent consilium.[111] The number of consilia in the collection is thus again much

107 di Gliozzi, "Capodivacca, Girolamo."

108 For more see Černý, *Mor 1480-1730*, 48; or Palmer, "Girolamo Mercuriale and the Plague," 51-65.

109 Capivaccius, *Opera omnia*.

110 Ibid., 4r. Epistola dedicatoria. "Quia vero … Pars practica, octo abhinc annis evulgata, denuo recudenda et ab adspersa Italorum Gallorumque Typographorum spurcitie repurganda erat …"

111 Ibid. This involves for example consilium XLVIII., under which in addition to that of Capivaccio, we also find the consilia of other renowned Padua professors Girolamo Fabrici d'Acquapendente and Alessandro Massaria. Similarly, e.g., 989-91, Cons. XLVII.; 991-3, Cons. XLVIII.; 956-8, Cons. XIII.

higher than the official figure. Collaboration between important professors was evidently not without difficulties, which is evidenced by Capivaccio's comment in one collective consilium: "...I assert that this medication will be absolutely useless."[112] Dates appear to a minimal extent and then only in the minutes of actual consilia with colleagues.[113] The names of patients are given sporadically, but they clearly show a clientele from the upper classes of society and from various countries (Paciens Gallus, Germanus, Polonus etc.). The first consilium, which clearly corresponds to one "history" at the end of the book, where an entire case is described in detail, is interesting.[114]

For comparison with the collections of the previous famous professors, a collection of a lesser-known figure was selected. Antonio Maria Venusti (Antonius Venustus, 16th cent.) worked as a municipal physician in Trieste. The biographical information we know is very modest, but so far, we know only that he was from a wealthy Milanese family and completed his studies of medicine in Bologna.[115] The fact that he was not among the absolute top physicians represented by university professors and the personal physicians of rulers is no reason to ignore his consilia. On the contrary, this offers an opportunity for a comparison of the approach to the genre of a physician with a lower but however not inconsiderable status. His "Consilia medica" was first published in print in Venice in 1571 during the lifetime of the author, who appears to have edited the collection.[116] Venusti dedicated his only work to the Habsburg Archduke Charles of Styria (1540-1590), under whose dominion Trieste belonged. In the preface "Ad lectorem," as the reason for the publication of his consilia, he mentioned the general need to receive assistance from others and because "of all tasks, the work of physicians is unanimously considered the most difficult..., for this reason in treatment even the most experienced physician must request assistance from other physicians in the form of their opinions and call them to consilium."[117] He

112 Ibid., 964-5, Cons. XX., "Ego.., assero, eam medicationem prorsus inutilem fore." Patavii. Besides the protesting Capivaccio, also signed by Bernardo Paterno, Girolamo Mercuriale and Girolamo Fabrici d'Acquapendente.

113 Ibid., e.g., 994, Cons. XLIX. Consilium in hernia ... medicorum subscriptorum, Patavii 20.11.1567; signed by "Aloysius Bellocatus et Petrus Zanonus-chirurgus;" 980-1Cons. XXXVIII. Besides Capivaccio, G. Mercuriale, M. A. Montagnana, G. Fabrici d'Acquapendente.

114 Ibid., 941-3, Cons. I. Pro patritio quodam Augustino; 997-8, Historia caussaeque obitus nobilis cuiusdam adolescentis.

115 Hirsch, *Biographisches Lexikon*, 86-7.

116 Venustus, *Consilia medica*.

117 Ibid., 4r. "... ex omnibus muneribus humanis munus medicorum gravissimum esse censeatur, ... quemlibet certe medicum vel peritissimum in merendo alios medicos consulere, in consilium

himself was purportedly called many times to consilia and by writing up cases wanted even more to "de humano genere promereri," and so make a contribution to subsequent generations. Most interesting is however the conclusion of the preface, where he described the order of the process to work on his 28 consilia. When writing them up, he strictly adhered to the three-part composition as outlined by authors Agrimi and Crisciani, and only dates are missing from an "ideal" consilium.[118] All mention the location of writing, names of patients and their social status. They also capture the "casus," regimen and medication in great detail. It seems that some consilia were written as the minutes of a meeting with colleagues.[119] Venusti's "customers" included patricians of various cities, but especially members of the archduke's court.[120] Nevertheless, neither members of the archduke's family, nor the Archduke himself are among the addressees of his consilia. Since this collection, because of the mention of complete titles and meticulous manner in which it is written up, including a brief summary on the margins, seems like an advertisement of a successful physician, the author certainly would not miss the opportunity to mention the names of such important patients.

The final author selected of Italian origin is Cristoforo Guarinoni (Christophorus Guarinonius, 1534-1604), a renowned diagnostician and language expert in Greek.[121] This native of Verona represents a kind of link or transition from the cisalpine consilia literature to that north of the Alps because he spent part of his life in Central Europe. Guarinoni completed his studies of medicine at the faculty in Padua under the guidance of above-mentioned professor Vittore Trincavelli with whom he remained in contact even after he completed his studies.[122] After completing his studies in Padua, he became the personal physician to the Duke of Urbino, Francesco Maria II. della Rovere from whose service he was lured away by the prestigious

vocare, aliorum medicorum sententiam exquirere oportet."

118 Ibid., 4v. "In plerisque vero hisce meis consiliis talem ordinem servavi [I kept this order]: primum de cuiusque aegri temperatione verba feci [I determined the patient's composition] ... deinde singulos morbos cum suis causis atque symptomatis diligenter consideravi [considered the causes and symptoms of the disease]: postea quibus in morbis opus fuit, prognosticum protuli [I made a prognosis]: postremo curationem morborum perscripsi [I prescribed treatment]."

119 Ibid., 57. "Cum alii multi morbi sunt, collegae doctissimi, ..."

120 Ibid., 1, Pro... patritio Mediolanensi; 46. Pro Ill. Georgio, comite ...; 210, Pro ... Principis Caroli ... Consiliario ac Regente electo ...; 144, Pro ... Principis Caroli Archiducis Austriae Consiliario et Cubiculario...; 152, Pro Ottobono Spinula, Patricio Genuensi ... etc.

121 For more about him see Divišová, "Ärzte mit den Nachnamen Guarinoni," 89-101.

122 Trincavellius, *Consilia medica*, 917. Epistola XXV.; 922. Epistola XXVI.

position of personal physician to Emperor Rudolf II. From 1590, his work is linked to the Imperial Court and Prague, where he also died. In addition to several philosophical and medical works, he also authored many consilia, which – how else – were published in Venice in 1610 after his death.[123] This book was edited by bookseller Paulus Meiettus, who also paid for its printing by typographer and publisher Tomasso Baglioni. Paulus Meiettus mentioned that the main reason for his actions was "an effort not to deprive humanity of the excellent results of this knowledge."[124] He dedicated the book to the famous Padua professor of medicine Girolamo Fabrici d'Acquapendente.[125] However, how Guarinoni's consilia got to Venice and why his consilia were not published during the author's lifetime, cannot be determined. One possibility is that the nephew of the author, Girolamo Guarinoni obtained the consilia from the estate of the deceased.[126]

622 consilia appear in the collection and even this high number was certainly not complete.[127] The names of patients and consulting physicians appear in approximately one third of cases and the same applies to dates and locations of the write up. The upper classes naturally predominate among the names of specified patients. At the time in which Guarinoni was active in his native Italy, the names of Italian nobles and patricians appear among his patients, and after he received the position as the emperor's physician, his services were sought after by those in high positions at the Imperial Court.[128]

123 Guarinonius, *Consilia medicinalia*.

124 Ibid., Ar: "...tanti viri scripta si hominum negligentia perirent, splendidissimo profecto lumine genus humanum destitutum dixerim, cum ... usum recte medendi humanis corporibus ostendat ..."

125 In addition to the dedication, the imperial privilegium, which ensured the publishing and copy rights, is worthy of attention; it was issued already on Jan. 1st 1601, and contrary to convention no time limitation is given for the privilegia, yet we do learn of the exact amount of the fine for its violation and a reminder of the duty to submit three copies to the office.

126 Hieronymus Guarinonius is "undersigned" on the physician's tombstone in St. Vitus Cathedral in Prague. For more see Hausenblásová and Šroněk, *Urbs Aurea*, 180. However, it is not certain that many of the consilia could not have been supplied by Italian friends and colleagues with whom Guarinoni was in contact. For more about the composition of the collection see Buršíková, "Sbírka konsilií," 23-38.

127 The collection is named Consilia, but the individual consilia are designated as "Consultatio." Several additional consilia can be found in both the unpublished collection of consilia for Spanish ambassador G. de San Clemente, which is in the care of the Strahov Library, as well as among the rest of Guarinoni's correspondence, preserved in the archive of the Biblioteca Oliveriana in Pesaro and in the Fondo Ducato of the municipal archive in Florence. The existence of more extensive correspondence is also evidenced by certain allusions in the consilia in which the author refers to a previous consilium, which however is not found in the collection.

128 In addition to members of the della Rovere family, members of the Gonzaga family, the Sforzas, as well as a range of cardinals and popes; in Prague for example the rector of the Jesuit

Many of the consilia were typical consilium-letters in which he responded to requests he received. In some such cases, he expressed dissatisfaction with the quality of the provided anamnesis.[129] Many consilia were evidently created ex post as a record of actual meetings between physicians. The names of then important representatives of the medical profession, both from among university professors and the Imperial Court, appear among the consulting colleagues.[130] More than a small number of consilia also "border" related genres because in their conclusions they include a commentary on the result of the case, most often however about the death of the patient and sometimes even with a brief post-mortem report.[131] Even in the case of Guarinoni, some records show that collaboration with colleagues was not easy.[132] With his activities in his native Italy and subsequently in Prague, Cristoforo Guarinoni represents the ideal link between the worlds of Italian and tramontane consilia literature, which was well received in German-speaking lands.

2.8 Representatives of Consilia Literature in German-Speaking Countries

Consilia literature flourished in Central Europe and the selected physicians represent only a fraction of the consilia authors. One important figure who cannot be omitted was Johannes Crato of Krafftheim (1519-1585).[133] After completing his studies of classical languages and theology at the

College, the Spanish Ambassador G. De San Clemente, the High Burgrave of Bohemia, alchemist Edward Kelly, or French Queen Elizabeth of Habsburg.

129 Guarinonius, *Consilia medicinalia*, 105, Cons. XCII. "To one of your letters ... I can reply briefly, but even so my consilium will not help her [the patient] very much because I have not been informed of many things that I need to define her illness."

130 Ibid., 39, Cons. XXX. On the French [disease] with G. Alessandrini, G. Capivaccio, G. Mercuriale and others. "This matter, wisest men and finest physicians, which was explained to us yesterday by a learned colleague ..." Similarly, e.g. 45, Cons. XXXII.; 295, Cons. XXVI etc.

131 Ibid., 190. Cons. CLXVII.; 489. Cons. CCCCXXX. "For ... Guilelmo, the Duke of Mantua... Three years later he died of it. When the corpse was opened, one kidney was completely destroyed ..."; 333, Cons. CCCXXX. To venerable Father Mario, Superior of the Capuchins...334 "He became cachectic, fell into fever and so died." The opposite result is recorded on 47, Cons. XXXII. "... he was healed, without consequences, and he married."

132 Ibid., 409, Cons. CCCLXXXVII. Consilium after a long disputation conducted against important physicians, especially Capivaccio concerning stomach problems ... of the noble V. Duke of Urbino, Guidobaldo II.; 353. Cons. CCCLI. "For the noble Duke ... a defense of the previous opinion ..."

133 Eis, „Crato von Crafftheim." For more see for example Evans, *Rudolf II and His World.*

University of Wittenberg, this native of the Silesian city of Wroclaw decided to pursue the study of medicine in Leipzig. From there, like many of his countrymen, he moved to the Mecca of medicine of his time, Padua, where he became a devoted pupil of the renowned Giovanni Battista da Monte. After completing his doctorate, he undertook a short trip around Italy, practiced in Verona and took the position of municipal physician after his return to his native city in 1550. Later, he accepted an offer to become the personal physician of Emperor Ferdinand I. and even remained at this post under his successor Maximilian II. Because of court intrigues connected with politics and religious antagonism, he encountered major problems at court after the ascension of the next emperor, Rudolf II., to the throne.[134] Despite this, he continued to be called to Rudolf during his health crises, so he was rightfully given the nickname "physician to three emperors." As one of the most educated humanists of his day, he represented a link between various intellectual movements and his correspondence documents contact with the most important European figures of the time.

Crato was the author and publisher of many expert medical works (recall the editions of da Monte's consilia), but his own consilia cannot be separated from the fate of Lorenz Scholz, a colleague over a generation younger. Lorenz Scholz (1552-1599) was born in Wroclaw, studied medicine in Germany and then Italy and subsequently practiced in Freistadt in Silesia.[135] He worked the greater part of his life in Wroclaw. He was one of the physician-natural scientists, devoted several years of work to botany and established a famous botanical garden in his native city.[136] His name and indisputable contributions are also linked to his publication activities. He became an enthusiastic collector and editor of consilia and the correspondence of both his contemporaries and predecessors, especially however of his admired countryman, friend and patron Crato of Krafftheim. Thanks to his activity, five collections and anthologies of consilia were compiled and published in Frankfurt between the years 1591-1594 under the name Crato of Krafftheim. Another two were published in Hannover in the year 1611, only after the death of Lorenz Scholz. We can also add one more anthology, compiled in the same spirit but on which Scholz did not bestow Crato's name, to this long list of publications.[137] The work on all these anthologies makes Scholz one of the most important editors of consilia in the German-speaking countries.

134 Gunnoe Jr. and Shackelford, "Johannes Crato von Krafftheim," 201-16.

135 Cohn, „Scholz von Rosenau."

136 For more see for example Oszanowski, "Wroclawski ogród," 99-102.

137 Scholzius, *Consiliorum liber singularis.*

Scholz dedicated the first book in memory of his friend Peter Monau, to whom belonged the published consilia and letters.[138] In the preface to "Ad sanioris Medicinae cultores Praefatio" the main reasons given for publishing the consilia were an effort to benefit humanity and remember the renowned figure of Johann Crato.[139] However, another reason mentioned was also patriotism, as documented by this call: "I ask the same of all, who are devoted to the medical profession, to kindly not refuse to provide me with any consilia written by German physicians, especially those, who have already departed, in which noble medicines or exceptional observations appear, especially since my efforts are directed at nothing but the glorification of physicians of our Germany and their commemoration for the future ... if I publish the received consilia, I will make a mention [about the providers] ..."[140]

In this collection, 28 undated consilia from Crato were published. Unfortunately, the names of patients were not mentioned at all. However, the manner in which they are titled, for example "Pro nobili viro," "Pro nobili puella" (For the noble sir, For the noble young lady etc.) indicates that the patients were from the upper classes. Consilia were evidently actually sent in the form of a letter, as can be concluded from various bits at the end. Publications of no-less-interesting medical correspondence were added to this and all subsequent collections.[141]

The second book was published just one year after the first and proves that Scholz's call to send consilia was not disregarded. The volume consisted of 30 consilia of six physicians, but only three of these spoke German.[142] The book was dedicated to another of Scholz's friends, the renowned Nuremberg physicians and humanist, Joachim Camerarius. In the preamble, in addition to repeating the main reason for publishing consilia – the public good (publica salus) –, the editor fulfilled his promise and thanked all those who had sent him consilia. In addition to several municipal physicians,[143] he especially highlighted the assistance from two important Wroclaw

138 Crato, Consiliorum liber. Monau came from an important patrician family in Wroclaw and was the court physician to Emperor Rudolf II. For more about Peter Monau see *Evans, Rudolf II and His World, 244*. Republication of this book from the year 1595 was dedicated to another of Scholz's friends, Severinus Gobelius, the personal physician to the Prussian duke.

139 Crato, Consiliorum liber, 2r.-3r.

140 Ibid., 4r.

141 This correspondence is treated at www.aerztebriefe.de

142 Crato, Consiliorum liber secundus.

143 Paulus Fridewaldus, Wenceslaus Raphanus, Iohannes Weidnerus, Petrus Rothus. Crato, Consiliorum liber secundus, 6.

humanists – Jacob Monau, the brother of the already-mentioned court physician, and Martin Weindrich, who translated the consilia sent to Scholz into Latin.[144] The author of the majority of the consilia in this anthology was Crato (21 consilia) with the rest split among: Johannes Neefe, the personal physician to Augustus, the Prince Elector of Saxony, two physicians to Emperor Maximilian II. and his son Rudolf II., Giulio Alessandrini and botanist Rembert Dodoens, another renowned botanist Pietro Andrea Mattioli and the Venetian physician Girolamo Donzellini. The names of the recipients of the consilia were again left out and dates were preserved for only five of them. References to the collection and exchanges of consilia even appear in the medical correspondence, which was published in the same volume. "Thank you greatly for sharing the consilia of Crato, copied down by your hand, and I will try to repay you in the same manner. I also have enough of them but have left them in Vienna. When I get there, I promise to copy them down for you as repayment."[145] Thus, physician Peter Monau promised his colleague Scholz to send Crato's consilia, and this even repeatedly.[146]

The third collection in many editions was published in the year 1592, shortly after the publication of the second.[147] It is evident that the German physicians were interested in public welfare as well as immortalizing their own names. Documentation of contact with renowned experts certainly served as good advertising for their practices. This time, Scholz dedicated the book to Salomon Albert, a professor at the faculty of medicine in Wittenberg.[148] In the preamble, where we will stop for a moment and which is dedicated to "all devoted to the medical arts," Scholz strongly supported the cataloging and sharing of consilia, especially in German-speaking territories:

> "Someone may wonder why I dare to publish so many consilia written by German physicians. ... Everyone knows that until now only the consilia of foreign physicians have been published. Our Germans have been satisfied

144 Crato, Consiliorum liber secundus, 5-6. This documents an effort to provide access to German consilia for the European scientific community and to obtain the widest possible clientele on the book market. For more on this topic see Maclean, *Learning and the Market Place*, 60, 66.
145 Crato, Consiliorum liber secundus, 368.
146 Ibid., 365. "I will make sure that all of Crato's consilia that I have are copied and I have already begun. I will try so that you do not receive too few, rather more, and just as good as yours." Ibid., 381. "I will send you Crato's consilium, which he wrote for me on this case, as soon as possible with the rest."
147 Crato, Consiliorum liber tertius.
148 Ibid., 2.

> with these and excessively admire them, while disregarding and skillfully concealing their own consilia even though they could benefit our people much more because medicine is practised completely differently in our country." And he added words aimed against competitor groups of healers to his arguments: "In other countries ... such a custom is observed that those afflicted by a disease ... turn to physicians and request their aid immediately after the illness breaks out. ... In our country, however, few consult with a physician immediately at the beginning of an illness and rather first try all folk cures ... and only request the help of physicians when the hope for life is minimal. ... Under these circumstances, who would not see usefulness of the application of these consilia, which ... directly teach what we must follow ...?"[149]

At the conclusion he emphasized how knowledge of consilia helps in the application of generally valid rules to individual cases.[150] He again repeated the same in the preamble to the fourth volume of the publication (see below). In this third volume, the editor tried a more systematic and scientific form of classification: consilia and their index are grouped according to the gender and age of patients into diseases of men and boys, diseases of women, virgins and diseases of girls (Morbi virorum et iuvenum; Morbi mulierum; Morbi virginum; Morbi puellarum) and the topic of each paragraph was added to the pages for convenience in searching. The anthology contains 38 consilia for patients from the upper classes. Almost half of the consilia (15) again are from Crato,[151] while the others are from ten other physicians. In addition to the famous, who need no introduction, such as Thomas Erastus, Theodor Zwinger, Johannes Aichholz, Giulio Caesare Aranzi, Caspar Hoffmann, Caspar Neefe and Helidoeus de Paduanis, there are consilia from lesser-known municipal physicians: Johann Sigismund of Schweidnitz and Joachim Cureus of Glogau. Worthy of attention is a consilium on which imperial physicians Hieronymus Stromaier and Peter Monau collaborated with Diomedes Cornarius, who also included the same consilium in his collection.[152]

149 Ibid., 2-5.

150 Ibid., 5. "...hanc etiam ob causam exercitatissimorum Medicorum observationes, quae praeterquam, quo modum universalia particularibus recte applicandi monstrant, plurima etiam ad graviores morbos remedia..."

151 However, two pseudo-consilia, which were supposed to contribute to prevention, are also included among his consilia. Crato, Consiliorum liber tertius. Cons. XVI. a general consilium on the Hungarian fever; Cons. XVII. an anti-plague consilium.

152 Ibid., 135, Cons. XXIX.

The fourth book of consilia was first published in the year 1593, only a year after the previous two.[153] Scholz dedicated it to the renowned physician Caspar Peucer, another of the personal physicians to the Prince Elector of Saxony, Augustus and concurrently a professor at the faculty of medicine in Wittenberg. In the preamble we find interesting motivations: a desire for knowledge, the great importance of medicine, and the usefulness of consilia: "... the difficulty lies most in the correct application of the general to the particular. It seems that consilia, which were prescribed for extremely complicated cases by the most experienced men in our arts, are best at this. Thus, I do not deserve censure for the desire that these consila sent variously by friends be accessible to inexperienced physicians..."[154] Scholz thanked many colleagues for providing consilia and unknown practical physicians appear among the famous names even here.[155] Even in this anthology the classification of consilia according to the age and gender of patients was followed, but this time only for "Morbi virorum et iuvenum" (diseases of men and boys) and "Morbi mulierum" (diseases of women). 34 consilia were published of which 26 consilia, again the majority, from Johann Crato.[156] Noteworthy is the "consilium" that illustrates the process of communication among the individual participants of the treatment process and mutual discrepancies. It untypically consists of four parts: the request for a consilium, which an unknown physician addressed to the professor from Padua G. Capivaccio, Capivaccio's consilium, the critical reaction to Capivaccio's proposed treatment from the physicians of the Bishop of Salzburg and finally the defense of the attacked G. Capivaccio.[157]

The fifth and last book of "Crato's" consilia edited by Scholz, was first published the following year in 1594 with dedications to the renowned professors of the faculty of medicine in Basel, Felix Platter and Caspar

153 Crato, *Consiliorum liber quartus.*

154 Ibid., 4.

155 The senders include the names of many practical physicians, who are essentially unknown today, such as: Achilles Croemer "marchionatus Moraviae medicus," Johannes Francus "physicus Camicensis," Mag. Iohannes Faber "Monsterburgensium et Francosteinensium Medicus ordinarius," and others. "Those most experienced," or those who were asked for consilia, in this book include, in addition to Crato, Abraham Seiler (Seyller), Caspar Hoffman, Andreas Gallus, and Caspar Neefe. The greatest thanks were in the preamble were expressed to the Wroclaw patrician Heinrich Schmidt, "who from the library of his relative, Abraham Seiler ... shared many useful documents." Undoubtedly, this refers to consilia. Crato, Consiliorum liber quartus, 5-6.

156 Ibid. Five consilia are dated, three are again "non-real" consilia with general applicability, e.g. 166, Cons. XXIII. De preservatione a peste.

157 Ibid., 135-57, Cons. XIX. In praeservatione et curatione podagrae, pro quodam nobili viro Salisburgensi.

Bauhin.[158] No preamble of the editor appears in this volume, so the suppliers of the consilia did not receive their rewards and advertising in the form of printed published acknowledgements. The division of the index of the consilia according to the age and gender of the patients into "Morbi virorum et iuvenum" (1-38) and "Morbi mulierum" (of which there are only two) remained unchanged. Of the total number of 40 consilia, Crato is the author of 34 and he collaborated on one with three other physicians.[159] The authors of the other consilia are Peter Monau, Iohannes Petrus Merenda of Brixen and Caspar Hoffman. What is interesting is Crato's last non-real consilium-treatise on women's illnesses before, during and after childbirth to which a regimen for the pregnant (a treatise on the correct health regimen during pregnancy) is attached.[160] This book concludes the continuous series of publications which was only resumed many years later.

The anthology of consilia, which this time Scholz published under his own name, also belongs in this series both conceptually and in the manner of editing. "Consiliorum medicinalium ... liber singularis" (The Unique Book of Medical Consilia), probably first published only a short time before Scholz's death, is dedicated to the Silesian Estates.[161] In the preamble, Scholz presented his efforts to the layman community thus:

> "... there exist two types of treatment. Either a physician, as appropriate, recognizes the nature of the illness, considers all circumstances and before all openly says what is necessary, ..., or he explains his opinion on the treatment and illness in writing and effectively also helps those who are far away. This second manner of advice is in our art correctly called consilium. ... The objectives of these consilia are two. In the first, we gratify someone far away, who has requested our opinion on his current health, while in the second, for chronic, long-lasting, and reoccurring illnesses we show, due to [our] experience, how to prevent and avoid new attacks of the illness."[162]

Something new and surprising also appears here: criticism of the consilia genre on the part of physicians, who refuse to make decisions regarding

158 Crato, Consiliorum medicinalium liber quintus.

159 Ibid., 239, Cons. XXXIV., signed by Johannes Crato, Nicolas Biese, Hieronymus Camutius [sic] and Thomas Jordan.

160 Ibid., 261-5, Cons. XL. De morbis mulierum ante partum, in partu et post partum; 265-75 Gravidarum regimen.

161 Scholzius, *Consiliorum medicinalium liber singularis.*

162 Ibid., 3r.-3v.

diseases based on what someone describes from far away – thus, without personal examination of the patient. The opponents of consilia placed the emphasis on personal "observatio et experientia" and supported their opinions by citing classical authorities Aristotle and Galen.[163] Scholz completely rejected any objections and explained the point of consilia in detail in seven theses. One of his most important counterarguments was the long tradition of writing consilia, which he proved with a list of authors from Baviera and Montagnana, to his contemporaries.[164] He further emphasized the role of the attending physician, who describes the illness and compiles information from consilia, thereby compensating for the personal absence of the counsellor. According to Scholz, the unanimous opinion of multiple physicians is decisive for proper treatment.[165] In his fifth counterargument, Scholz mentioned the existence of consilia, which are not intended for patients, but for convalescents or those concerned about a certain disease, thus preventative consilia.[166] To refuse someone requesting a consilium in his view means to leave a patient completely at the mercy of a disease and also a colleague "high and dry." He did not forget the importance of consilia for the education of students, for the general health and benefit of the scientific community.[167] The ten-page preamble from "Liber singularis" represents not only a unique period epistemological definition of the consilia genre with its types, designated purpose and evaluation of significance, but also captures the stages in which the medical community under the influence of the growing importance of neo-Hippocratic trends also admitted even the darker aspects.

After this short detour, let us return to a listing of the names of physicians and laymen, thanks to whose contributions, Scholz was able to compile "Liber singularis." The forty names of the authors include professors of famous

163 Ibid., 3v. Cited are Aristotle's words "those, who decide based on few indicators, are easily mistaken" ("qui ad pauca respicient, facile fallantur") and the opinion of Galen, who refused to advise an epileptic boy remotely because he had never seen him.

164 Ibid., 4r. "... numquam tamen rationes istae, vel si plures etiam sint, tantum valuerunt, ut Medicos superiorum aetatum, ac nostro quoque a Consiliorum utriusque generis communicatione absterrere potuerint."

165 Ibid., 4v.-5r. "...plerique, in quorum gratiam alibi consilia conscribuntur, Medicos suos, a quibus omnia, quae ab absentibus ordinantur, rite gubernari possunt, domi habere solent."

166 Ibid., 4v. "... quo multa consilia non amplius aegris, sed vel convalescentibus, aut iis, qui morbum aliquem metuunt, ut praservationi contra morbos inserviant, praescribantur."

167 Ibid., 5v.-6r. "Consilia ... aliis etiam Medicinae studiosis, qui ea legerint ... non dubito profutura cum aut publicae hominum saluti consulerem; tum ut studium meum bene de multis promerendi posteritati teratum facerem, liberali pectore communicare volui ..., ac Reipublicae literariae modis omnibus gratificandi cupidissimo, profesa sunt: ..."

faculties of medicine (e.g., G. Rondelet, J. Sylvius, G. Capivaccio, T. Erastus, et al.), personal or court physicians of ruling families (J. Crato, G. Alessandrini, A. Vesal, A. Seyller et al.), and today lesser-known municipal physicians and practitioners (J. Baudis, B. Schneider, M. Ratzenberger, P. Sybellenus et al.). In total 383 consilia were published in the anthology. These were divided into parts on diseases according to age and gender like "Crato's" three previous collections.[168] As however the editor himself noted, not all were published for the first time. However, re-edited consilia from previous volumes were "supposedly significantly amended and improved."[169] The editor carefully marked 220 original consilia with a star. Scholz claimed that 50 of these were from Crato. For unknown reasons, two of Crato's medical works were added before the series of consilia,[170] while following the edited consilia a treatise on by the physician Caspar Hoffmann on spas,[171] two of Crato's treatises on fevers and the plague,[172] and finally Capivaccio's manual for correct cauterization,[173] were also added, which caused the work to grow to monumental proportions.

For understandable reasons, among the authors there are the names of many physicians connected with the imperial court: Crato, Monau, Alessandrini and Dodoens. It is worth a short detour away from the topic to note that the anthology also contained ten first-published consilia from the pen of a professor of the University of Montpellier, Guillaume Rondelet;[174] and others were published in the sixth book of "Crato's" consilia (see below).[175] If such a large number of consilia of a French physician were found in German-speaking countries, it would be surprising if it were not possible to find others in France. We can only wonder (not for the last time) why no printer or devoted student, who would publish the consilia of such a well-known figure separately, could be found.

168 Morbi virorum et iuvenum 304 consilia; Morbi puerorum 15 consilia; Morbi mulierum 55 consilia; Morbi virginum – three consilia; Morbi puellarum sive consilia.

169 Scholzius, *Consiliorum medicinalium liber singularis*, 4r. "Elenchus consiliorum...quorum ea, quae asterisco sunt notata, ac numero suo prius edita longe superant, plane nova ac rara ...: Reliqua vero antea quidem sub Doctoris Iohannis Cratonis...nomine a me evulgata fuerunt. Verum editio praesens priore multo emendatior et locupletior, nonnulorum quoque locorum restitutione melior..."

170 Ibid. "Mikrotechné, seu parva ars Medicinalis" and "Analogismus, sive Artificiosus transitus a generali methodo ad exercitationem particularem." Without foliation.

171 Ibid., 1061-68.

172 Ibid., 1069-157.

173 Ibid., 1158-64.

174 Ibid., the first number designates the consilium and the second the page. 39/108; 90/235; 108/290; 123/338; 193/566; 197/574; 233/687; 293/837; 304/871; 349/975; 305/873; 325/920.

175 Five consilia were printed here.

Now we come to the final two volumes published under Crato's name. The sixth and seventh volumes were published in Hannover after the death of the founder of the series, L. Scholz.[176] Despite this, surprising references about his contribution to their compilation, which evidently do not correspond to the truth, appear in the titles of both publications.[177] Both publications lack dedications, but Scholz's preamble, which is identical to the preamble of his "Liber singularis"[178] appears in the sixth book. The sixth book includes 109 consilia. The largest number (28) again belong to Crato, but many of his consilia had already been published in previous collections and the same applies to several consilia of another twenty physicians.[179] Eighteen consilia lack a clear designation of the author, which besides the incorrect numbering contributes to the impression that the publication was prepared rather carelessly. Medical correspondence was also added to this volume of consilia.

The seventh volume is analogous to the sixth: it was published in the year 1611 in Hannover and like the previous collection also lacks dedications and a preamble as well. The index is followed by an extensive treatise from Crato of Krafftheim,[180] and furthermore by 106 consilia from 21 authors, most of whose names we know from the previous collections. They again include important Italian, French and German professors of medicine and personal physicians of noble courts as well as lesser-known representatives of the medical arts.[181] The new editors used the consilia of Johannes Crato (29) and Girolamo Capivaccio (20) to the greatest extent. Among Capivaccio's "consilia" we find a republished record that appeared under the title "The History and Causes of Death of One Noble Youth" in his "Opera omnia,"[182] or

176 For more concerning the details and circumstances of the move of the heirs to the renowned printing company of André Wechel from Frankfurt to Hannover in the year 1597 see Maclean, *Scholarship, Commerce, Religion*, 100.

177 Crato, *Consiliorum liber sextus*; Crato, *Consiliorum liber septimus*.

178 Crato, *Consiliorum liber sextus*: "Ad Lectorem aequum et candidum proemium." 6r. Datum Vratislaviae in Aedibus nostris, die 26. Martii, Anno salutiferi partus 1598.

179 For completeness, I am including the names of all persons: M. Acacia, J. Baudis, G. Capivaccio, J. Crato, M. Curtius G. Donzellini, C. Hoffmann, J. Neefe, G. Neefe, H. de Paduanis, B. Paterno, J. Ratzenberger, H. Reserus, G. Rondelet, V. Schoenfeld, B. Scheider, A. Seyller, H. Stapedius, M. Stoiius, P. Sybillenus, J. Sylvius, A. Vesal.

180 Crato, *Consiliorum liber septimus, Analogismus, sive artificiosus transitus a generali methodo, ad exercitationem particularem*. The pages of this treatise are not numbered in the publication, but one can say that it contains 165 pages.

181 For those interested, I have included the names of the physicians concerned: A. Bottoni, G. Capivaccio, J. Crato, G. Donzellini, A. Fracanzani, A. Gallus, C. Hoffman, P.A. Mattioli, J. Neefe, G. Neefe, J. Pfeil, M. Philippus, G. Rondelet, J. Sigismundus, I. Schaller, B. Scheider, A. Schurfius, A. Seyller, J. Sylvius, J. Tagaultius, S. Weiskopf.

182 Crato, *Consiliorum liber septimus*, 30-5, Cons. VIII.; Capivaccio, *Opera omnia*, 997-8, Historia caussaeque obitus nobilis cuiusdam adolescentis.

the republished dispute between Capivaccio and the physician of the Bishop of Salzburg, which was recorded in the fourth of "Crato's" collections.[183] The only novelty in "Crato's" seventh collection is an effort to place consilia regarding one specific disease together. Thus, in this publication we find consilia on the treatment of podagra from Rondelet, Crato, Seyller and Capivaccio,[184] grouped together and we also find the same approach for other diseases such as the treatment of sterility.[185]

A really detailed analysis of all the above-mentioned collections would certainly provide far more information. In summary, one can say that of the first five volumes of "Crato's" consilia, only the first is a collection, while the other volumes, including Scholz's from the year 1598, are anthologies to which several dozen physicians contributed their consilia. In total, 390 consilia, designated by the editor as completely original, were published here and Crato is the author of 146 of them. This enumeration does not include the two Hanoverian anthologies, which were only published by Wechel's successors without the participation of Lorenz Scholz.

After a rather extensive analysis of Scholz's monumental series, we will now focus on Crato's younger contemporary Reiner Solenander (Gathmann 1524-1601) from Büderich by Wesel.[186] He first studied medicine in Leuven, but from the year 1549 started to travel around the Italian faculties of medicine in Bologna, Rome, Naples and Pisa, where he was a student of the renowned but quarrelsome professor G. Argenterio, into whose disputes he entered significantly as his defender.[187] He even managed to attend several universities in France. He started his career as a physician at the sulfurous spa in the Italian city of Lucca, but after his return to his native land in 1559, he accepted the post of personal physician to Duke Wilhelm V. (1539-1592) of the House of Jülich-Kleve-Berg, which he held for almost 40 years. As a friend and colleague of physician Johann Weyer, an opponent of witch trials, today considered one of the founders of psychiatry,[188] even he fought against superstition, exorcism and the persecution of witches. Solenander became the author of several works. His work on sulfurous springs, which put him among the pioneers of balneology, brought him exceptional fame. His only

183 Crato, *Consiliorum liber septimus*, Cons. XXIV.; Crato, *Consiliorum liber quartus*, Cons. XIX.
184 Crato, *Consiliorum liber septimus*, Cons. XXVII.-XXX.
185 Ibid., Cons. XC.-XCII.
186 Dieckhöfer, "Solenander, Reiner."
187 For more concerning the figures and disputes between Giovanni Argenterio and the personal physician to Emperor Maxmilian II. Giulio Alessandrini (Iulius Alexandrinus) as well as Solenander's role in the dispute, see Siraisi, "Giovanni Argenterio," 351-4.
188 Binz, "Wier, Johann."

purely medical work is a collection of consilia, the first part of which was already published in the year 1558. The complete work was published after Solenander's "retirement" in the year 1596.[189]

He dedicated his complete edition to his lords and employers, the Dukes of Jülich.[190] In the motivation mentioned in the first edition of his consilia, he gave valuable testimony about the popularity of consilia at the time and how random their publication could be:

> "… my friend J. F. de Gabiano was supposed to publish in print the famous consilia of Montanus and when he saw that the book was not achieving befitting dimensions, he asked me to add any in the event that I had in the course of treatment obtained and kept any. I thus agreed and gave [him] some, which he added, and although I knew that I am an inexperienced novice, it was even so liked by many so much that the copies were easily taken, and none was left at the booksellers. Because I promised in my publication to later add some others [consilia], it happened that many physicians from various locations accosted me almost daily with pleas and calls to publish them if I have any, and if I [were] not yet finished with them, to provide the book printer with at least the first edition, which was published in 1558, sold out and unavailable."[191]

On the following page, in the preamble to the readers however Solenander emphasized that the main reason for publishing his consilia was "in gratiam medicinae candidatorum."[192]

The collection is split into five parts, which include a total of 136 consilia. Patients naturally came from the upper, more affluent classes.[193] Their names

189 Reinerus Solenander, *Consiliorum medicinalium sectiones quinque, quarum prima ante annos triginta octo … Lugduni edita cum consiliis … Joannis Montani in 16 excusa. Reliquae quatuor ab autore iam recens additae* (Francofurti: apud Andreae Wecheli heredes, 1596).

190 Ibid., 2.

191 Ibid., 2r.-2v. "… amicus meus J.F.de Gabiano, … Montani celebria consilia sub typis haberet excudenda: videretque, quod liber iste in iustam magnitudinem no excresceret, me rogavit, ut si forte quae excepissem in curationib.meis, atque servassem, ea istis addeerem. Consensi tum et dedi quaedam, quae addidit. Ea licet rudis ego et tyro notassem: plauerunt tamen multis, ita ut exemplaria facile distraherentur, neque iam ullum apud Bibliopolas exemplar prostaret. Quoniam vero in mea editione promeseram, me porro alia paulatim additurum> factum est, ut multi ex diversis locis Medici [2v.] pene quotidianis precibus et hortationibus, contenderent, ut si qua haberem, communia facerem. Vel si illud integrum non esset, saltem primam editionem (quae anno 1558 facta et iam distracta non inveniretur) Typographo concederem."

192 Ibid., 3r. Solenander Medicinae studiosis salutem.

193 Ibid., e.g., 20, Cons. V. Pro Ill. quadam Comitissa; 71, Cons. XVIII. Pro mercatore Florentino; 80, Con. XX. Ad mercatorem Nurembergensem; 198, Cons. XXVII. Wilhelmo, Comiti a Schwartzenburck…

are mentioned sporadically, which is somewhat compensated for from the standpoint of historians by the numerous names of attending physicians, the consilia of some of whom were also presented in Solenander's collection (anthology). No matter how much Solenander pronounced the great demand for his consilia before readers, certainly neither their recipients, nor their attending physicians came from the highest circles of power. His renown is however attested by the fact that those interested in his consilia included not only physicians and patients from his native Germany, but also from countries in which he studied, especially from Lucca and Lyon, as well as from Spain and England.[194] Multiple consilia are clearly just supplementary records made after consultation with other physicians.[195] In addition to cooperation with individual colleagues, Solenander also collaborated with municipal medical associations.[196] Dates appear on about one third of his consilia with a lesser number dated in the 1560s and 1580s, while a greater number are from the 1570s and 1580s.

Compared to other authors, Solenander included a large number of "request" letters of his colleagues in the anthology. In one of these requests for a consilium, Solenander was explicitly asked by the attending physician to come and participate personally in the treatment. The patient allowed for advice in the form of a letter only as an alternative option explicitly under the condition that he send an instructed physician, proficient in both anatomy and surgery, with the consilium.[197] Among the interesting cases was a "consilium," however designated as a "historia" concerning a female patient, who had hallucinations and wanted to fly. Solenander sent this case to his friend Johann Weyer as a specialist in this area.[198]

194 Ibid., 121, Cons. VII. Ad D. Ludovicum Perez Hispanum, ... ult. Octobri, Anno 84, Hambachi; 113, Cons. pro Ill. Domina Angla, ad Excell. Doct. Waltherum Baylaeum in Angliae Oxoniensi academia medicinae professorem.

195 Ibid., Cons. XXI. Pro ... cive Lucensi, habitum cum Medicis Genevensibus.

196 Ibid., 5, Con. II., In vertigine pro cive Lucensi ad Antonium Minutolum Lucensem Medicum; 181, Cons. ad D. Petrum Spinam Doct. Medicum; 15, Cons. IIII. Pro mercatore Argentinensi ... Affectus qui hunc virum, expertissimi medici, iam longo tempore male habuit ...; 66, Cons. XVI. In calculo... ad Fabricium nobilem Lucensem medicum...

197 Ibid., 235, Sectio III., Cons. VIII. Scriptum D. Schelii, de affectu ... viri Georgii Duicker, ...ad Reinerum Solenandrum. "Aeger, mater ipsius, amita mea, nosque omnes tuam praesentiam petimus et flagitamus [...we all long for your presence]. Quod si propter urgentia tua negotia, quod etiam aulicis curis impediaris, fieri haud possit [if you are not able to come], rogamus, ut exercitatum in anatome et chirurgia Medicum, vestro consilio instructum, qui tutissime et foelicissime Medicinam faciat, ad nos quamprimum mittas [send a doctor who is versed in anatomy and surgery with your instructions] ... 29.5.1576." Solenander's response was sent on June 1st of 1576 from Cleves.

198 Ibid., Sectio IV., 322, Cons.VII. Item de Virgine ... historia describitur ... Iohanni Wiero, praeclaro viro atque humanissimo. Lemgovii, Idibus febr.1568.

Another selected author of consilia was Diomedes Cornarius (1535-1600), who was born in Zwickau to a much more famous father.[199] Diomedes studied medicine in Jena, Wittenberg and Vienna and contrary to the custom of the time evidently never attended any Italian university. In the preamble of his consilia, he mentioned that he practised several years in Trnava "in Ungarn," in order to earn money for his doctoral graduation. He graduated in the year 1568, joined the staff of professors at the faculty of medicine in Vienna and eventually became the personal and court physician of the emperor's brother, Archduke Maximilian of Habsburg.[200] "Consiliorum medicinalium ... tractatus," first published in the year 1599, is his only work.[201] It is not entirely clear whether Cornarius lived to see its publication and his work was published at the expense of the bookseller. He dedicated his work to Archduke Maximilian and as the reason for publication mentioned (unsurprisingly) the effort to help students of medicine and already practicing physicians. In the preamble, he warmly thanked a person well-known to us, Lorenz Scholz, who published several of Cornarius's consilia in Crato's anthologies and thus gave him the impulse for his own publication.[202]

The rendition of the entire work is rather unusual. Although it was published under the title "Consiliorum tractatus," Cornarius (or an unknown editor) also included independently numbered "Observationes," "Historiae admirandae rarae," and several of Cornarius's ceremonial speeches.[203] Of the 20 consilia, only one half are actual consilia, while the rest rather resemble "observations." As an illustrative example of how these genres overlap, one can present two classic consilia intended for an abbot, written one year apart by the same physicians, which are supplemented by a description of the cauterization performed on the patient, which is designated as the third "consilium."[204] Other "consilia" record the results of treatment, occasionally even with a description of a pathological autopsy,[205] while again some rather resemble theoretical treatises.[206]

199 See Hirsch, "Cornarius, Janus."

200 Hirsch, *Biographisches Lexikon*, 80.

201 Cornarius, *Consiliorum medicinalium tractatus*.

202 Ibid., 1.

203 Ibid., A2.

204 Ibid., 101, Cons. XII., dated August 1st 1583; 123, Cons. XV., dated May 20th 1584; 126, Cons. XVI., dated December 10th 1584.

205 Ibid., 73-4, Cons. VIII.

206 Ibid., 83-9, Cons. X. De loquelae defectu cum surditate. This is a description of the medical history of an 11-year-old boy to which an extensive analysis of the general causes of deafness and its treatment has been attached. G. Pomata, who however focused more on Cornarius's "Historiae," called attention in her work to the epistemic significance of this thorough and

Cornarius is specific with respect to the chronology and thorough dating of consilia (as well as observations) written from the 1570s to 1590s, even regarding the names of physicians who participated in the cases.[207] Among those colleagues named, there are mostly municipal physicians, court physicians from German ducal courts, and also several physicians connected with the imperial court, for example Bartholomeo Guarinoni, Ottaviano Rovereti, Peter Monau, and others. The identities of patients were not revealed, but from titles it is evident that they were from the highest classes, but there were also exceptions.[208] Individual consilia are long and detailed and Cornarius didn't leave out any of the three components of consilia. Like all graduated physicians, not even he avoided denouncing references to competitor healers.[209] The sixth consilium, which even includes the "request" letter, is worth mentioning. Surprisingly, the author of the detailed Latin description of symptoms in the "request" letter was not the attending physician, but the husband of the patient. He also asked Cornarius to see to the messenger and purchase of medicines at the pharmacy.[210]

Thomas Mer mann (1559-1622) is another of the German physicians who contributed to the spread of consilia literature. He was born in Cologne into a wealthy family, and completed his studies of philosophy of Pisa, where he then successfully lectured. He also completed his studies of medicine there and returned to his native land with a doctorate, where he worked for several important nobles as a personal physician. In this post he finally put down roots with the Dukes of Bavaria, who even utilized him as a political advisor and diplomat.[211] Mermann's "Consultationes ac responsiones medicae" were published half a century after the death of this important physician by a

chronologically ordered dating of consilia, observations and histories. For more see Pomata, *Praxis historialis*, 105-46.

207 Cornarius, *Consiliorum medicinalium tractatus*, 20.

208 In the consilium dedicated to the treatment of a child with dysentery, we however surprisingly find "Pro pauperibus medicinae," which includes many prescriptions for the treatment of dysentery from ingredients financially affordable even for the poor. Cornarius, *Consiliorum medicinalium tractatus*, 27-30, Cons. II., 31-46.

209 Ibid., 39. "... in multis dysentericis, quod ab Empiricis Iudaeis absque ratione male curatos [treated improperly by Jewish empirics] ... dum doctorum Medicorum consilia aspernarentur ... Nec vero Iudaeos solummodo hic notare volui, sed etiam Christianos utriusque sexus homines ... [... but I must also blame Christian empirics]"

210 Ibid., 64-5, Cons. VI.

211 Due to his loyalty to them, he even refused an offer to become the personal physician to Emperor Rudolf II. Because of the above-mentioned services that he performed for the Bavarian lords and who certainly counted on Mermann's employment at the Imperial Court, it is possible that the refusal came from the other party.

professor of medicine and author of consilia, F. I. Thiermair, who we can thank for Mermann's biography.[212] His father, also a professor of medicine, Thomas Thiermair, was Mermann's guide and apprentice in his final years and it is also likely thanks to him that many of Mermann's consilia survived.

The title page of the collection already says everything important about the editor's work: he collected consilia "with great zeal from variously scattered manuscripts" and arranged the translations of parts of consilia from German and Italian into Latin and augmented them with replacement medicines and notes.[213] The work was dedicated to the Bishop of Eichstadt, Marquard and was published at the expense of the printer. In the preamble "Ad Lectorem," the editor again left us several details regarding his work:

> "I collected these consilia from various manuscripts here and there either randomly purchased, or borrowed from friends, or kindly sent to me from elsewhere. Many renowned men contributed ... In the meantime, it was determined that our Mermann, famous among scholars, rulers and their archiaters, composed and gave many more, even countless medical responses, which until now are hidden in various hands. Mermann allegedly often complained that difficulties with letters and just copying take up almost the whole day. Because Mermann mostly dictated the already mentioned letters in German and haste to his assistants (it never occurred to this exceedingly good man, to whom all glory was foreign, to publish such writings in print for the public), I first had to translate them into Latin, organize and arrange them into books. I corrected flaws, if any intruded by fault of time or negligence of copiers, and I admit that, as a person very busy with other work, I hated this activity. However, so the reader knows, which responses Mermann dictated in German or Italian and thus were translated by me into Latin, I have marked them all ... with a star."[214]

Although the words in the preamble belong to a physician living several generations later, there is no doubt that most anthologies and collections of consilia were created in an analogous manner. Under these circumstances, Thiermair published 219 consilia of Thomas Mermann, divided into eight

212 See Gerabek, "Thiermair, Franz Ignaz."

213 Mermannus, Consultationes ac responsiones medicae, Ingolstadii: Typis Joannis Phillippi Zinck, 1675.

214 Ibid., 6r.-v.

books according to the type of disease.[215] Most often we find actual "advice from afar," but even records belonging to the "historiae" genre appear.[216] The exact dates and locations where consilia were written are often given, but the specific names of patients appear sporadically. From the titles used it is evident that patients again were from the upper classes, including representatives of the houses of Habsburg and Hohenzollern, or the famous Fugger family.[217] Most of the dated consilia naturally fall within the period, when Mermann was already famous and respected, and were written starting in the 1580s usually in Munich, while the latest bears the date of 1612.

The first consilium where an editor's note appears at the end, is noteworthy and proof of the selective choice of printed consilia. The editor notes that the physician of the patient wrote back the following month to inform about the course of the treatment and asked about the next steps. Mermann answered with another consilium, but this correspondence was not included in print.[218] Occasionally, an editor notes that some parts of consilia were not preserved, usually prescriptions that were then added according to other prescriptions for similar illnesses from Mermann.[219] He evidently occasionally communicated directly with patients.[220] Several "request" letters have also been preserved in the collection and the most interesting of these is Mermann's request for a consultation from a colleague

215 Ibid., Liber primus de morbis capitis, hujusque partium (35 consilia); Liber secundus de affectibus faucium, colli et pectoris (21 consilia); Liber tertius de ventriculi et intestinorum vitiis (32 consilia); Liber quartus de hepatis ac lienis partiumque vicinarum accidentibus, praecipue de affectionibus hypochondriacis (43 consilia); Liber quintus de renum, vesicae ac genitalium incommodis (30 consilia); Liber sextus de mulierum morbis (18 consilia); Liber septimus de malis externis et cutaneis, nec non articulorum doloribus (33 consilia); Liber octavus de febribus (7 consilia).

216 Ibid., Lib. I., 52, Cons. XVI. Delirium cum furore in juvene nobili. Ad medicum quendam. "Cum nuper hinc discederet serenissimus archidux Ferdinandus, reliquit apud nos juvenem, qui ..."

217 Ibid., Lib. I., 84, Cons. XXVIII. Oculorum affectus pro Serenissima Archiducissa. Ad medicos ordinarios. Monachii 1609; Lib. III., 212, Cons. XXII. Pro Ill. comitissa...; Lib. IV., 238, Cons. I. ... pro ... Archiduce Ferdinando ... Ad Philippum Menzelium Medicum Professorem Ingolstadiensem ... Monachium 1591; Lib. V., 356, Cons. VIII. Renum calculi ... pro quibus Ill. Baro ... Marcus Fuggerus remedia petit ...; etc.

218 Ibid., Lib. I., 1, Cons. I., Porrigo capitis ... pro virginie nobili ... Monachii 1587, 4. April; 6, "NB. Eodem anno, mense Maii, rescriptum a medico ordinario, hanc curam esse peractam ... Responsum est a Mermanno ..."

219 Ibid., Lib. I., 41, Cons. III. "NB: In hoc Consilio defuere medicamenta ... Interim tamen spero, ea fere me substituisse, quae Mermannus alias in similibus praescribere solitus est."; likewise ibid., 44, Cons. XI.

220 Ibid., Lib. I., 48, Cons. XIV. Melancholia cum ... pro quadam foemina conjugata. Ad Maritum Virum honestum. "Ad ea, quae de uxore tua scribis, ..."

for himself.[221] Although most certainly consist of letters-responses to the written requests, several times Mermann expressed dissatisfaction with "advice from afar."[222]

From Catholic Bavaria, we now continue on to our next physician in Lutheran Saxony-Anhalt. Joh annes Wit t ich (1537-1596) was born in Weimar, studied medicine in Jena and Vienna, after completing his studies practised in Sangerhausen and Eislenben, and even worked for some time as the physician of Count Mansfeld-Vorderort. In 1578, he became the personal physician to the Counts of Schwarzburg and concurrently worked as a municipal physician in the Thuringian town of Arnstadt. He is the author of several works about natural science and medicine; however, he wrote mostly in German.[223] His anthology of consilia also contains the correspondence and "request" letters of other physicians and was published posthumously under the care of his son.[224] In the introduction to the work, dedicated to the Prince Elector of Saxony, Christian II., the editor highlights the contributions of his father, who tried to help the suffering despite his own serious illness.

> "My father was so diligent that he kept true accounts of not only his own cases, but also recorded and sought out the consilia of other excellent physicians from all over with all his strength for the sole purpose of settling the account of the wealth entrusted to him, not to keep them secret at home, but to one day share them with the public. He started to translate consilia from German to Latin, which after his father's death was finally completed by M. Erasmus Hedanus."[225]

The reason for collecting consilia was thus supposedly, as for others, to bring relief to the sick and to try to improve medical knowledge. Like other physicians, here consilia were translated into Latin only because of publication and the work was published at the expense of the bookseller, not the son. Worth a marginal mention is the comment of Wittich junior in the dedication, where he captured a memory of the grandfather of his patron, the Prince Elector of Saxony, Augustus, who "… tirelessly refined the most noble and never sufficiently pronounced hermetic philosophy and

221 Ibid., Lib. IV., 300, Cons. XXVIII. "Hypochondriaca aliaque graviora, quae ipus Mermannus perpessus est, symptomata. Ad Henricum Boterum Medicum. Monachium 1600."
222 Ibid., Lib. VII., 500, Cons. XVI. "De affectu cruris, a reverendo patre Mario in schedula breviter descripto, sine autopsia recte judicare est difficile, …"
223 l. u., "Wittich, Johannes."
224 Wittichius, *Medicorum consilia.*
225 Ibid., 3v.

medicine, which is called chemistry."[226] It is evident that Wittich Jr. not only approved of this attitude, but also gave it as an example.

Besides the name of Johann Wittich, the following list mentions another 20 names of exclusively German physicians who contributed their consilia. Three of them cannot be identified and evidently belonged to the circle of less important municipal physicians.[227] However, more numerously represented are the names of renowned representatives of the German "Res publica medica."[228] The anthology includes 80 consilia, letters and observations and is not divided into genres. Dates are given very often, while the location of their writing and names of patients, who according to their titles came from the wealthy classes, appear less frequently.[229] The name of professor of medicine and the first rector of the university in Jena, Johann von Schröter (1513-1593), who also worked as the personal physician of the Duke of Saxony, Johann Fridrich II appears frequently among the counsellors. 34 consilia, almost half of the entire collection, are from this physician. The reason why Schröter himself or his students or descendants never published these consilia independently remains unknown.

From among the large number of variously approached consilia, six consilia and three letters, the subject of which is the health of one patient, are noteworthy.[230] The author of the first has not yet been identified, while another three consilia are evidently from ordinaries from the hometown of the patient. The third consilium is remarkably detailed. The individual articles of the six "res non naturales" are analyzed in separate treatises. Despite this, the patient was not satisfied and requested the advice of another physician to whom he evidently provided the previous consilia. In three separate letters, the new counsellor criticized the opinions of his colleagues and replaced them with his own consilium. Although we failed to determine

226 Ibid., 4r. "... nobilissimam et nunquam satis commendatam hermeticam philosophiam et medicinam, quam chemiam vocant, indefesso studio excoluit ..."

227 E. g. M. Taurerus, O. Maroltus, G. Tinskerus.

228 The physicians listed below were professors of faculties of medicine or the personal physicians of the German temporal and ecclesiastical aristocracy: G. Von Andernach, I. Brambachius, A. Ellinger, T. Erastus, B. Grünewaldt, G. Marius, G. Oetheus, J. Pontanus, S. Wilde, J. Willichius. More bibliographical information about these historical figures can be found at www.ärztebriefe.de.

229 Wittichius, *Medicorum consilia*, 9, Cons. II. "... pro generoso quodam comite"; 521, Cons. LXXII. "... pro quodam Cancelario Mansfeldico."

230 Ibid., 107, Cons. XIII. ... pro quodam Rectore Scholae Isleb. Ordinatum a clarissimo viro D. D. Matthaeo Ratzenbergero, Medico praeclaro; 112, Cons. XIIII. D. D. Simonis Wilden in eodem affectu pro eadem persona; 114, Cons. XV. Alterum D. D. Simonis Wilden; pg.116, Cons. XVI., Tertium pro eadem persona ordinatum a D. Simone Wilden, Physico Islebiano tunc temporis; 128, Cons. XVII. D. Doctoris Pontani pro eadem Persona; 137, Cons. XVIII. Sequuntur quaedam epistolae medicinales Pontani ad praedictam personam. (written in Gotha, dated the year 1556, three the year 1557).

the identities of the participants, the file well documents the competition for customers within one profession and at the same time illustrates the options that a patient could select. In the following consilia there are also many interesting details, which would deserve closer analysis and evaluation, and, like all consilia collections, would also merit a separate detailed study.

The last German author that this work covers, Johannes Matthaeus, was selected because of his distinctive approach to the anthology and reasons for its publication. The link in fact became the treatment of one patient.[231] Neither Matthaeus's personal data, nor his fate in life are known, but thanks to references in his work, we know that he was the last personal physician to Margrave Ernest Fridrich of Baden-Durlach (1574-1604). After the death of his master in the year 1604, he continued his career as a municipal physician in Hannover and later as a professor in Singen in Baden. In addition to the above-mentioned book, he is also the author of a treatise on the Baden spas, which he published in the same year as his anthology of consilia.

His work was not dedicated to any important figure, which is exceptional compared to other authors. The preamble for readers, which begins with the description of the manner of treatment "per analogismum" among the Egyptians (supposedly from the pen of the classical historian Strabo) and an analysis of a more scientific approach to treatment based on Hippocrates and Galen, is for the greater part devoted to the denunciation of dabbling in medicine.[232] Right at the beginning, Matthaeus clearly presented two main reasons for publishing the consilia:

> "... So that all would recognize the foolishness [of dabblers] and at the same time to comply with the requests of many physicians, who still now desire to learn what disease our faithfully departed ruler suffered from and what the opinions of physicians of the time regarding it were. So, my work is published, and it captures which consilia were written at various locations for the noble lord and all came together in my hands with which though unworthy I led the lord's treatment ... I even attached the "secrets" of some empiricists, so that disseminated foolishness and lies are dispersed like clouds, evident contradictions of dabblers, childish nonsense, old wives tales and finally dangerous experiments ... could be shown ..."[233]

231 Matthaeus, Consilia medica.
232 Ibid., 1r-3r.
233 Ibid., 3v.-4r.

A record of the treatment of the patient, administered medicines and even the names of most of the physicians and healers who spent time at the side of the ruler during the final six years of his life, follows. Various "Anabaptists," Jews and transient healers supposedly surrounded his lord, who suffered from various problems for 8 years, and promised recovery for a great payment. The work was thus clearly published as a defense of the correctness of treatment by university-educated physicians, especially by the editor himself. The objective was to clearly point to those responsible for the death of the patient and avoid any suspicion of his own failure.

The editor collected nine consilia in the collection. Of these, he only wrote one himself, three are from professors at the faculty of medicine in Heidelberg, three are from personal physicians of important nobles, one is evidently from a paracelsian physician, and one is even from a Spanish theologian.[234] However, Matthaeus's commentaries also include the names of other more or less well-known physicians, who were even in the slightest manner involved in the treatment of Ernst Fridrich, for example the renowned Felix Platter.[235] All of the consilia are precisely dated, were created between the years 1599 and 1601, and even include the locations that they were written or sent from. The editor of the anthology ordered the consilia chronologically and wrote a detailed analysis and evaluation for each. The worst evaluations were given to the alchemy-oriented paracelsian Balduinus Clodius and "Franciscus Bornius Hispanus de Madrigal Theologiae doctor," whose dabbling was denounced by Matthaeus by means of a derisive couplet.[236] The actions of dabblers, who evidently received significant sums of money from the patient, are mentioned continuously throughout the entire work.[237]

234 Doctors deserving of a mention are Petrus de Spina, the personal physician to the Prince Elector Count Palatine of the Rhine, and Iacobus Mosanus, personal physician to Moritz of Hessen. For more on the significance of this figure see Salloch, *Das hessische Medizinalwesen.*
235 Matthaeus, Consilia medica, 142. "Ceterum eodem anno [that same year] cum Clarissimus Medicus Felix Platerus Durlachum transiret et Cels. sua officcii caussa salutaret [... when Felix Platter passed through Durlach ...], inter alia remedia, quae in deliberationem veniebant, mentio fiebat [among the drugs that were possible, he also mentioned] ..." For more concerning the visit of Felix Platter see Baumann, "Ernst Friedrich."
236 Matthaeus, Consilia medica, 32. "Fingunt se Medicos quivis Idiota, sacerdos; Effrenis Monachus, plenaq[ue] fraudis anus."
237 Ibid., 87-8. "... iudaeus quidam commendatione comitis cuiusdam Rhenensis se insinuaverat, qui certis characteribus auro inclusis mirandos promittebat effectus, insignis et urinarum inspector haberi volebat ..."; 105. "Longum esset, ..., omnium, qui empirici haberi volunt, nugas et vanitates hic commemorare, quas tamen multi tantopere Ill. Principi hoc tempore commendabant ... Ante alios erat quidam sexagenarius, natione Gallus nomine Theodoricus rerum naturalium

After the consilia and commentaries, the editor surprisingly added one more contribution "Ad lectorem," where he published the consilium "written by the hand" of Italian physician Girolamo Donzellini, who was among the physicians connecting parts of Europe in religious strife by means of information.[238] In his closing epilogue, Matthaeus (in addition to presenting other prescriptions for the treatment of podagra from other famous physicians) just simply stated that Ernst Friedrich died on April 13th 1603 at the age of 44 years of a catarrh associated with his previous podagra.[239]

2.9 Representatives of French Consilia Literature of the 16th Century

The first French representative is a contemporary of Montanus and Trincavelli, Jean François Fernel (Ioannes Fernellius, 1497-1558), who needs no introduction. During his lifetime, through his numerous works, he gained a reputation as one of the most important reformers of Galen's teachings.[240] His life was linked primarily to Paris, where he completed studies in philosophy, mathematics, astronomy and of course medicine, which he also taught there starting in 1534. He eventually became the personal physician of Henry II. of Valois and his wife Catherine De Medici. The combination of his post at the university and position as the personal physician of the ruler brought him great wealth and renown, and many physicians turned to him with requests for consilia. There were supposedly over four hundred of Fernel's consilia among his acquaintances.[241]

A selection of Fernel's consilia was first published in 1582 after his death under the care of his student, the Parisian physician and professor, Gillaume Capelle. Capelle dedicated the work to his older colleague, Julien Le Paulmier, as thanks for not refusing to provide Fernel's consilia for publication,

plane imperitus, ...;" 106. "... quidam Thomas Rhetus ... insolentior factus Illustrissimo Principi sub pretio vel remuneratione 2000 flor. suam operam addicebat..."

238 Ibid., 120. "Medicae artis tyronibus rem gratam me facturum putant, si hisce Germanorum medicorum consiliis pro podagra conscriptis Itali, ... medici Hieronymi Donzellini, de eodem morbo iudicium, quod manu ipsius Auctoris conscriptum habeo, subiicerem ..." For more about Girolamo Donzellini and his significance see Quaranta, "Exile Experiences," 74-6.

239 Matthaeus, Consilia medica, 127. Historians who wrote about the life of this noble naturally did not devote attention to medical works. Thus, for example W. Baumann, the author of the most detailed biographical study of Duke Ernst Friedrich von Baden-Durlach, determined, concerning the illness and treatment of this noble, only that in 1600 Ernst Friedrich took some physician from the Prince Elector into his service. Baumann, Ernst Friedrich, 173.

240 For details see Deer Richardson, "The Generation of Disease."

241 Fernellius, *Consiliorum medicinalium liber*, 1582.

"although he could keep them as a treasure."[242] However the impulse for the publication of Le Paulmier's "epitome" was not only respect for Fernel, but also an effort to contribute to public welfare.[243] Concerning his editorial work, Capelle said that he neither added nor removed anything and only translated some things from French into Latin.[244] He also apologized for his less neat writing style.[245]

The number of published consilia is not high at 70 and five request letters.[246] For several consilia, the complete request letters were not printed, only their concise excerpts.[247] Only eight consilia are dated, all from the 1550s, at the end of Fernel's life and period of his greatest renown. Most patients were left in anonymity, though several of the mentioned names disclose a clientele not only from among the highest French nobility, but also from abroad.[248] The 29th consilium captures both the cooperation of physicians as well as the moving story of a female patient. Here, the attending physician turned to colleagues who had successfully treated his patient in the past.[249] In the anamnesis, he

242 Ibid., a II r. "... a te tibi ex innumeris adversariis quae curae tuae commitebat, ut eius editionem mihi ... demandares, cum potuisses tanquam thesaurum relictum ab eo tibi servare." Julien Le Paulmier (Palmarius 1520-1588) was among Fernel's devoted students and followers of Fernel's teachings.

243 In the second edition of the consilia the reasons for publication were expanded to include the assistance of studying youth and patients. Fernellius, *Consiliorum* liber, 1585, 3r. „... iuniorum conatus iuvare possint, illa etiam publicae luci committere et aegrorum valetudinem fide et scripto immortali restituere ne differas."

244 Fernellius, *Consiliorum liber* 1582, a II v. Eight consilia and one request letter were translated from French.

245 Ibid., a III r. "Ne ... eius orationis familiarem qrandiloquentiam hic quasi demissiorem appare: cum enim Epistolae quaedam sint et extemporanea consulta humiliorem stylum ex composito et decoro requirere videbantur."

246 De facto there are 71 consilia since 2 consilia were mistakenly designated as number 13. Republications from the years 1585, 1589 and 1597 were augmented, yet still always only contain around eighty consilia. For more on the reprints of Fernel's works and details about the publications of consilia see Sherrington, *The Endeavour*, 187-207.

247 In the second edition of Fernel's consilia all of these concise "anamneses" were called "Historia." In the first edition, this designation rarely appears, for example, in the request letter of the physician Claudius Melinus. For details see Fernellius *Consiliorum liber* 1582, 8r.-8v. Cons. 6. Pro Nobili virgine; 8v.-9r. request letter: Historia morbi praecedentis scribente et interrogante Claudio Melino.

248 Ibid., 16r., Cons.12. Responsum D. Fernelii ad litteras D. Du Perat in aula caesarea viri percelebris seu Medici eius Bucheri; 79v., Cons. 39. De febre quartana. Pro Regina Leonora; 83r., Cons. 43. ... Pro Domino de Maligny; 24r. Cons. 13. [falso] Pro D. Alberto Iuniori Marchione Brandemburgensi; 68r., Cons. 34. Pro Cancellario Imperatoris Caroli V., etc.

249 Ibid., 60r., Cons. 29. Pro comitissa Alesiorum. Rescriptum eius Medici. „... sedulitate atque diligentia vestra liberatam audio (Viri Doctissimi). ..."ibid., 60v. „... non modo a vobis evicta, sed etiam totius corporis constitutio melior multo quam ante morbum effecta est. "

described the development of her state of health, several premature births and miscarriages of the patient and their treatment in detail; followed by a consilium prepared by Fernel and his colleague.[250] Also unique is a consilium that begins with a request sent to Parisian physicians, continues with the response and concise information about the death of the patient and her autopsy.[251] Fernel's consilium on the case is inserted separately at the end.[252]

The last consilium that I would like to call attention to is the request of physician Cornelius Melinus concerning a consilium for himself.[253] This likely involved an important representative of the medical community. According to references in consilia, he treated quite important figures.[254] The reason for "bothering" Fernel, for which he very politely apologizes at the beginning, was a difference of opinion among physicians regarding his treatment, specifically strong bloodletting, which Melinus vigorously resisted with references to Galen.[255] Fernel's response documents his stance on this classical authority.

> "You have fallen into ... the doubts, which have tortured the souls of almost everyone, who intended to do medicine and devoted himself to scientific activities and practice. That [doubt] stemmed from Galen's works. There is such a diversity, such a volatility, and for the most part such a disunity that hardly anyone arrived at a decision concerning this thing ..., but not even he, if I may judge concerning this contentious question, ever firmly decided in favor of anything certain and consistent since [93v.] he devoted his entire life rather to thinking than the manner of treatment. Here, I would not act as an interpreter, nor would I try to

250 Ibid., 61v.-62v. Responsum Domini Fernellii et D. Du Mouceau.

251 Ibid., 39r.-41r. Rescriptum Domini Crabe Medici Regii ad Medicos Parisienses, Pro Domina De L'aubespine [sic], Tabem minante; 41r.-42r. Cons. 20.

252 Ibid., 42r.-43r. D. Fernellii scriptum, dum desserendum illi esset cum aliis Medicis aulicis De affectibus Dominae Del'Aupespine [sic] ... 1553.

253 Ibid., 91r.-93r. Litterae D. Melini Medici Ad Dominum Fernellium, De sanguinis missione in pruritu. „Quae negotiorum tuorum sit magnitudo, quae item molestiae, non ignoro: omnes enim qui graviore aliquo morbi genere laborant ad te non aliter quam ad Aesculapium quendam confugiunt:.."

254 In the second edition of the consilia, there are more letters from Dr. Melinus, for example, for the Marquis de Sablé. Fernellius, *Consiliorum liber* 1585, 24v.-25r. Littera D. Melini ad Fernellium Pro D. de Boisdauphin etc.

255 Fernelius, *Consiliorum liber* 1582, 91v.-92r. "... iterum aperui basilicam ... Chirurgus autem quem mea cuassa Claudius Lavallus Regis christianissimi Legatus vocaverat et medici in ea erant sententia, sanguinem multum esse vacuandum. ... Sed ego Galeni sententiam sequutus..."

> decide about completely contradictory statements of the author, but what I would consider through long practice as if learned, I would explain … with several true statements [theoremis], which would completely rid you of the awakened fears …"[256]

Of course, Fernel was very well acquainted with Galen's work, as he demonstrated at the end of this consilium:

> "Everything certainly agrees with what you took from the 4th book „*De sanitate tuenda*". Contradictory statements follow that which Galen orders in the 3rd book „*De locis affectis* …" And he overconfidently concludes it all with a reference to his own opinion and work: „But all of this is rejected by us, and the previous decision supported in the book that we have called „*De vacuandi ratione*." I will do no more because I am variously occupied by many different activities. …"[257]

Although the 16th century was a time during which Galen's work was undergoing re-evaluation together with criticism, Fernel's stance on Galen and his work could have been considered by many people as practically heretical. This stance together with the brevity even brusqueness of most of his consilia, without a plethora of references to authorities and citations from their works, which were common in the consilia of Italian physicians, could have resulted in the not completely positive reception of Fernel's consilia by the academic community.

The second and final French physician of the 16th century who became the author of consilia collections is Fernel's student Guillaume de Baillou (Gugliellmus Ballonius, 1538-1616). De Baillou was born in Paris and apparently also spent his whole life there. It is not known whether he took a study trip elsewhere. He graduated from the faculty of medicine in Paris in 1570, and then successfully split his career between service at the royal court of Henry IV. of Navarre and teaching at his alma mater. In the years 1580-81, in addition to the position of professor, he also held the post of dean at the faculty of medicine.[258] He died at the ripe old age of 78 as a wealthy and respected citizen.

256 Ibid., 93r.-94v., Cons. 46. Responsum Domini Fernellii ad Dominum Melinum super quaestione proposita.
257 Ibid., 93v.-94r.
258 For details see Lonie, "The 'Paris Hippocratics', 155-74.

During his lifetime, he only published a pamphlet against surgeons demanding autonomy within the framework of the faculty. His most important works, especially one regarding epidemics,[259] including three books of consilia, were published posthumously between the years 1635-1643 under the care of his nephew, physician Jacques Thévart. Through comparisons of these works, historian I. Lonie proved that they were created concurrently with the consilia between the years 1570-1574 and pointed out interesting parallels.[260] In individual consilia, references to cases mentioned in the book on epidemics, or in "histories," which were published in the third book of consilia (see below) even appear.[261] The reason, why de Baillou did not publish the consilia himself, is "a mystery" according to I. Lonie because he evidently intended to publish and had prepared a dedication.[262] For the first book of consilia, de Baillou, as was the custom, wrote a preamble to the reader (Ad lectorem), and this was already in the year 1572.[263] At the beginning of his second book, for some unknown reason, one can find two preambles, both dated to the year 1575.[264] For the third book of consilia, de Baillou apparently did not leave an address for the readers, and so instead of this, Thévart used a letter that de Baillou had designated as the preamble to another work.[265]

However, as editor for the first book, Jacques Thévart wrote a no less interesting introduction, where he uncovered the important motivation for the accelerated publication of the consilia. He determined that other than the important physician Jean Fernel, no French colleague had published a work of this kind.[266] The other reasons for the publication of the consilia are not very surprising: "to learn an easy method for treating highly numerous and unprecedented diseases, which are more frequent in Paris than among

259 Thanks to these works, de Baillou is considered one of the precursors of modern epidemiology.
260 Lonie, "The Paris Hippocratics," 172.
261 E.g. Ballonius, *Consiliorum liber secundus*, 218, Cons. XII.
262 Lonie, "The Paris Hippocratics," 169.
263 Ballonius, *Consiliorum liber primus*, 1635) 31-4.
264 Ballonius, *Consiliorum liber secundus*, without pagination. Benevolo lectori, 23.11.1575; Admonitio ad lectorem ... 15.11.1575.
265 Ballonius, *Consiliorum liber tertius*. "Haec epistola ex libro Epistolarum Medicinalium Ballonii nondum edito excerpta, praefigi debet libro de convulsionibus, anno 1640 edito." A letter is addressed to the ruler's archiatrus Myron in which Ballonius expresses his gratitude for his admission among the personal physicians by the King. Unfortunately, nothing more is known about the fate of the unpublished collections of Ballonius's medical correspondence.
266 Ballonius, *Consiliorum liber primus*, 8. "Quod ne mihi probro adscriberetur, ex omnibus Ballonii operibus editioni paratis, quorum me ille heredem testamento instituit, Consilia haec medica primum in lucem emittenda censui, quo scilicet a plerisque Philiatris desiderari, nullaque doctissimorum Collegarum (excepto Fernelio) ea de re scripta opera exstare animadvertim."

other nations"[267] and an effort to contribute to the medical community.[268] It is also worth mentioning the attempt of the editor to justify his changes to the consilia, such as leaving out certain parts and adding his commentaries to the Greek, and apologise for the fact that the consilia are not ordered "from head to heel" (a capite ad calcem), which was common for works on practical medicine (practica).[269]

The three published collections of de Baillou's consilia contain a total of 294 consilia: 119 consilia in the first book, 52 in the second and 123 consilia published together with 8 histories (historiae) in the third. Many consilia include dates as well as the names of patients, among whom one can find not only persons of high social status, for example, the secret advisor to the king, many nobles and their family members, as well as patients from among merchants.[270] Most of the identifiable names testify rather to the French scope of de Baillou's fame with the capture of only a few interested parties from other European countries.[271] Even de Baillou's consilia were intended rather for the hands of the patient's attending physician. Because of this, we sometimes also learn the name of the relevant colleague.[272]

French faculties of medicine, professors and instruction were among the best in Europe, although the development of medicine took a different

267 Ibid. "Primum enim perfectam facilemque addisces methodum medendi plurimis morbis inauditis et curatu difficillimis qui in hac florentissima Parisiorum urbe, propter frequentiam et celebritatem, saepius quam alibi gentium aut sanandi, aut dijudicandi proponuntur: ..."

268 Ballonius, *Consiliorum liber tertius,* a II r.-v. "Quae hactenus e musai nostri latebris in apertam lucem prodiere Clarissimi Ballonii opera ... ea tam gratiose ac comiter ab omnibus philiatris excepta sunt, certo ut credam peccaturum me in Remp. Iatricam si reliqua, quae adhuc latent, eiusdem authoris monumenta diutius apud me retineam ... medicinalium consiliorum, paradigmatorumque centurias aliquot ab ipso Ballonio iam seniore conscriptas mihique pronepti concreditas..."

269 Ballonius, *Consiliorum liber primus*, 9. "... quae superflua mihi visa fuerunt multis in locis subtraxi, scholiaque aliquot passim iis quae ex Auctoris peculio sunt adjunxi." The need to add an explanation to the original citations of Greek authorities confirms the assumption of I. Maclean concerning the poor knowledge of Greek among physicians. For details see Maclean, *Logic, Signs*, 19-20.

270 Ballonius, *Consiliorum liber primus*, 11, Cons. I. ... Ad Dominum Andream Guillardum, Regium in Consilio Secretiore Consulem; Ballonius, *Consiliorum liber secundus*, 200, Cons. XLVIII ... Pro Consule Tholosano; etc.

271 One of the exceptions, see for example in Ballonius, *Consiliorum liber tertius*, 215, Cons. I. "Anglus annos natus 46..."

272 Ballonius, *Consiliorum liber secundus*, 183, Cons. I. ... Ad D. Jaulnay Medicum. Even the final note "Cetera tibi tua singularis et eruditio et diligentia suppeditabit." (Your unrivalled knowledge and meticulousness will help you resolve the others.) testifies to the previous claim. Likewise ibid., 272, Cons. XXXVII. De Causo pro D. de Torigny. Ad Dominum Dalibourg Medicum Senonensem.

course than in Italy. This difference is clearly evident in the genre of consilia literature: in the course of the 16th century, only Jean Fernel lived to see this.

2.10 The 16th Century Consilia Literature – Summary

In the previous chapters, attention was devoted among other things to the status of physicians on the theoretical professional ladder, circumstances around the publications of their consilia and interesting information found in dedications and individual consilia. Let us now briefly recall the facts that have been learned.

Of the six selected Italian physicians of the 16th century, only two – Venusti and Guarinoni – were not connected professionally with the academic world and the other four, Vettori, da Monte, Trincavelli and Capivaccio, were important professors of medicine at the universities in Bologna and Padua. Except for Capivaccio, all had experience with running a municipal practice, to which however only Venusti remained faithful, while for Guarinoni the post of a personal physician was typical, and the primary role of the rest was teaching. Most consilia from the collections are understandably from the period of the greatest fame of each individual. Nevertheless, it was evidently not unusual to send a request for advice to a faculty, not to a particular professor.

Only two – Vettori and Venusti – could influence the publications of their consilia because they were printed during their lifetimes and in both cases the publications were financed by important Venetian printers. Publications of the consilia of the four others occurred after their deaths, mostly after a very long period of time. Da Monte's and Capivaccio's consilia were published 40 years, Trincavelli's 18 years, and Guarinoni's only six years after the years of their deaths. The initiators as well as most of the editors were in the cases of da Monte and Capivaccio their German students, Trincavelli's son took care of his first publication, and in Guarinoni's case an important book printer showed diligence, which also applies to the second mentioned publication of Trincavelli's consilia. If changes were made to the text or translations, editors made an effort to inform readers of their changes to the text.

If based on dedications we evaluate the reasons for the publications of consilia, we find that the most frequent motives, at least according to how they were declared, were efforts to benefit all of society, contribute to humanity and help others, as expressed in the preambles of J. Crato, H. Beyer and the bookseller Meiettus, who were behind the publications of da Monte's, Capivaccio's and Guarinoni's consilia and the same objective was also mentioned by Venusti. The second most frequently mentioned reason was respect and admiration for a professor, which Crato and Beyer immortalized, or the son's love of Bernardo Trincavelli. The oldest, Vettori moreover highlighted the benefits of consilia since they best capture the particulars of a given location and its inhabitants and the disease and treatment connected with them. In addition to these motivations, one can easily think of others such as financial benefits or obtaining certain advantages. As an example, we can use the publisher Valgrisi, who dedicated the collection of Venusti's consilia to the physician P. A. Mattioli as thanks for his recovery, but also remembered to thank him for entrusting his other works to his print shop. The printer Waldkircher dedicated Trincavelli's publication of consilia to the famous Danish physician Severin in order to draw his attention to the potential services of his Danish friend. For authors who published their consilia during their lifetimes, one can expect their desire for publicity, for advertising, which is however the case with only two of the six mentioned physicians – Vettori and Venusti.

Even though according to the titles of the volumes of consilia discussed, one could conclude that each physician was the author of his collections, a detailed examination reveals that the works of the Paduan professors da Monte, Trincavelli's second publication and Capivaccio's are rather anthologies. On the preparation of individual consilia, they either collaborated for example with other members of the faculty (Trincavelli), or other professors expressed their opinions on a case by means of their own written records (Capivaccio). Thanks to this collaboration, captured in the anthologies mentioned, we can expand the group of Italian authors of consilia to include additional names (Falloppio, Bellocati, Landi, Fracanzani, Frigimelica, Fabrici, Massaria et al.). The number of consilia in individual collections and anthologies varies significantly, but precise enumerations and comparisons have no point because of the randomness of the inclusion of consilia in a printing and our inability to factor in quantitative increases in reprints of consilia collections, as the publishers themselves already draw attention to them on the copyright page for advertising, and because of the fact that like Capivaccio's collection, one consilium can hide many others underneath. The lowest numbers of consilia mentioned in collections are found in Venusti's (28) and Vettori's (44). All are however outdone by Cristoforo Guarinoni with 622 consilia. Even hundreds (da Monte 434, Trincavelli 249, Capivaccio officially 51) appear in anthologies, but as already mentioned, the authors were always several physicians.

The composition of individual consilia is very diverse. A three-part composition was only strictly followed by the oldest, Vettori, and the youngest, the municipal physician Venusti, of the selected authors. Although they lag far behind their countrymen in the number of consilia, their emphasis on adhering to the traditional parts of consilia and the meticulousness with which they prepare individual entries go beyond the others. It is possible that their personal participation in the publication, which the others did not have, played a role here. The form of the anthologies and individual consilia was of course influenced by the approach of the editors and for the consilia of university professors (especially for da Monte's consilia) even the meticulousness of attentive students. Guarinoni's consilia are particular not only in that it is not clear by whom and how they were recorded, but also by the tendency to utilize consilia for a very long scientific, authority-citation-loaded treatise, which rather resembles a tractate.

Names of patients, exact dates and locations in which consilia were written are more the exception, but nevertheless thanks to the mentions of titles, it is evident that the absolute majority of patients were from the wealthy classes of society. The exception that proves the rule was da Monte, whose students at lessons in hospitals also wrote consilia-consultations for poor persons. This is also confirmed by the well-known fact that posts of municipal physicians usually attracted local notables, while professors of renowned Padua had a higher-level clientele and moreover even from abroad. The highest status patients can be found at the personal imperial physician, who also collaborated with the Paduan professors.

The selected representatives of consilia literature from German-speaking countries came from a politically and religiously diverse region, which however had no influence on either the approach to consilia, or the treatment process. If we disregard the practical inseparability of the figures of Crato and Scholz, seven physicians have been included in the selection. If we focus on their concise biographies, we determine that all but three figures – Cornarius, Wittich and Matthaeus – made use of the opportunities of peregrination and enriched their knowledge at various Italian universities, while Solenander even experienced the faculties of French universities. A clear majority of them started their professional careers in the role of a municipal physician. Only Lorenz Scholz remained in this position, while the others advanced to more highly recognized (and better paid) positions of personal physicians to more or less important German courts or nobles. Crato however achieved goals completely incomparable with the rest. On the other hand, only one of the selected representatives, Diomedes Cornarius tied his fate to the academic world.

If we look more closely at the published consilia works, we find that an absolute majority of them are anthologies. Although one author, editor or printer handled their collection and publication, dozens of more or less important physicians from various countries contributed their consilia to them. Only Mermann's collection and the first collection of Crato's consilia can be called true collections. As with the Italian authors, consilia were mostly published only after the deaths of their authors. This is the case of Crato, whose consilia were collected and edited by his friend Scholz not long after Crato's death. Mermann's consilia were published half a century after his death by the son of Mermann's intern, while the consilia of J. Wittich were edited by his son and published ten years after his death. The collections or anthologies of the other physicians (Solenander, Cornarius, Matthaeus) were published during their lifetimes. At least three works, by Cornarius, Mermann and Wittich (and evidently even the last two volumes of "Crato's" consilia), were published at the expense of printing houses and booksellers.

The reasons given for the publication of consilia will not surprise us in any way. In the first place is an effort to contribute to the public welfare (publica salus) or the scientific community (res publica litteraria), as expressed by Lorenz Scholz, furthermore, an effort to assist physicians in difficult decisions concerning the treatment process (Solenander, Cornarius), or to help students of medicine (Cornarius). These are followed by love of one's father and an effort to honor him with the publication of his work (Wittich), while completely new is a defense against accusations of malpractice and a fight against dabblers in medicine (Matthaeus). However, even here one must also assume undefined reasons: efforts of self-promotion, confirmation of one's position in society and not least the financial benefit, which certainly played a role for publishers and perhaps also for descendants. In the publications of consilia anthologies, at whose inception stood Lorenz Scholz, the preambles contain one more interesting aspect, which we do not find elsewhere: an effort to obtain and publish exclusively consilia written by his countrymen. The reasons are justified by the particulars of regional diseases, but here a role was played by a struggle against a sense of inferiority with respect to Italian medicine.

Most dedications of collections and anthologies are intended for the patron or employer of the relevant author or editor. Scholz however dedicated his works to friends from the medical community, mostly to members of the staff and professors at important German faculties of medicine. The number of consilia in individual collections and anthologies varies greatly from only nine in Matthaeus's anthology to several hundred in most of the others, to which however many other physicians contributed knowingly or unknowingly. The names of twenty contributors appear in Wittich's anthology, and the situation is similar in Scholz's publications.

Let us remember that Crato's consilia are only found in the first collection, and between six and ten physicians always contributed to the rest. 40 contributors even appear in an anthology published under Scholz's name. The consilia of many professors, who taught medicine and never published their consilia independently, were published in these anthologies. These include renowned physicians like Heidelberg professor Thomas Erastus (1524-1583), Basel professor Theodor Zwinger (1533-1588) and Jena professor Johann von Schröter (1513-1593).

It is noteworthy that many of the selected representatives of German consilia literature are only represented by request letters in their collections and anthologies. This applies to the collections of Cornarius, Mermann and to an even greater extent to Solenander and Wittich. Request letters, which are important for understanding the entire case and are more common in consultation literature of the 17th and 18th centuries, are understandably not found in the anthologies edited by Scholz or Matthaeus because their approach to and objective of the entire work were different.

With regards to the social status of patients, it also applies here that they came from the wealthy classes. Due to the large number of authors, it is often impossible to determine the status of physicians-counsellors, but we can with certainty say that J. Crato had the highest status patients. Unfortunately, no consilium has yet been found for any of the emperors he treated.[273] Other physicians with very important clienteles were Mermann, Solenander and Cornarius, which confirms that the position of personal physician to a high-status noble served as a good calling card and recommendation. Based on the occasionally preserved dates of consilia, one can estimate that all the physicians involved were the most requested counsellors during the peak of their professional careers (for example, Mermann in the 1580s and 1590s, Cornarius in the 1570s and 1590s, etc.). Crato, whose Central-European renown and popularity continued even after he left the limelight, was the only exception.

And now we come to the only two French representatives of consilia literature: both were connected to Paris, both taught at the faculty of medicine there, and at the same time both held the position of personal physician to the French Kings. Due to this, their patients came from the highest classes and in the case of Fernel there are even several high-status

273 However, worth a mention is a part of one of Crato's letters in which the formula of a mixture that he evidently used in the treatment of one of the emperors is given. For more see Crato, *Consiliorum liber quintus*, 43, Epistola X. "Hanc quoque sequentem misturam memini S. M. Pragae profuisse."

patients from surrounding countries, which is missing in de Baillou's consilia. The collections of the consilia of these physicians were published posthumously, in both cases over 20 years later. A devoted student was behind the printing and publication of the consilia of Jean Fernel, while de Baillou's were published by his nephew. The reasons for publication, which the editors mentioned in the introduction, are not uncommon but for one exception. G. Capelle, who took care of Fernel's consilia, mentioned respect for his teacher, an effort to help students and benefit the public and health of the sick, while the reasons in the preambles compiled by de Baillou were professional. However, in his preambles beside the expected love and respect, his nephew, J. Thévart added several more factors: he emphasized the suitability of consilia for instruction, their illustrative nature in the treatment of particular local diseases, an effort to benefit the "Res publica iatrica," but especially to enrich the scientific library with a genre on which no-one in his native land with the exception of Fernel worked.[274]

Fernel was the author of one collection of consilia and de Baillou authored a total of three. It should however be emphasized that in their cases, these were actual collections, not anthologies. De Baillou is the clear victor with regards to the number of published consilia (almost three hundred consilia), but according to the claims of Fernel's students, Capelle and de Paulmier only a selection of his four hundred manuscript consilia was published. Why only a maximum of eighty were submitted for printing (even republications) and what was the fate of the others is a mystery. This lack of clarity is even reinforced by a reference in a letter which the important Central-European humanist Andreas Dudith sent to his friend.[275] "Now, if you have not yet seen it, [I am sending] you at the same time together with [the works of] Donzellini, Fernel's consilia, which I have not yet read, but only glossed over. But as they seem worthless to me when I compare them with da Monte's.[276] ... The whole of Fernel's work is supposedly being compiled again in Paris with the additions of many things and at least four hundred medical consilia."[277] This news was either mistaken, or the realization never happened.

With this commentary from Dudith, we bid farewell not only to J. Fernel, but also to the other 15 selected physicians and their literary works. In this

274 This is a confirmation of the assumptions of historians who deal with consultation literature of the 17th-18th centuries. For more see chap. 4.2. of this work.

275 For more about this figure see Smolka, "Hájkův přítel," 125-168; or Almási, *The Uses of Humanism*, 239-363.

276 Crato, *Consiliorum liber tertius*, 313.

277 Ibid., 313-15. Andreas Dudith ab Horekouiza etc. Wenceslao Raphano Med[ico] ... Breslae [sic], 19 Iunii, anno 1583.

not particularly entertaining section, the circumstances, which influenced the genesis of individual consilia and collections and without which it would not be possible to comprehend a range of connections, were intimated. Some conclusions will again be applied in the synthesizing section that is devoted to consilia literature and the scientific community of the early modern period.

2.11 An Outline of the Development of Consilia Literature in the 17th and 18th Centuries

Consultation literature did not disappear from the literary market, but rather enjoyed popularity until the end of the 18th century. Certain changes occurred naturally, but the fundamental principles of consilia or consultation literature remained unchanged. Some of the trends introduced into our genre by developments in society and the natural sciences in the 17th and 18th centuries are worth mentioning. A more detailed study based on the biographies of physicians and the detailed analyses of their collections or anthologies would be almost unbearably tedious, so we will focus on only a few observations.

From the mid-1600s, the practical experience of physicians grew in value, while the number of publications of all types of specialized literature that recorded actual medical cases increased. The number of physicians who actively participated in the affairs in "Rei publicae" by recording and publishing procedures from their practices, continued to increase. The number of graduates from existing faculties of medicine gradually increased, while at the same time new universities were being established, some even in outlying parts of Europe. Not only the personal physicians of the nobility, university professors, but especially "mere" municipal physicians and lower status surgeons engaged in professional discussions within the framework of the scientific community and began to share their experience to a greater extent. In his work, Jena professor of medicine W. Rolfinck (d. 1673) characterized the statuses of 76 of those requesting a consilium in the following manner: "... some [of them] hold eminent positions and enjoy the titles of doctor and licentiate, and some are renowned practitioners."[278] A significant impulse

278 Rolfincius, *Ordo ... continens Consilia medica*, C2v. "Nomina Dnn. Consultantium, qui partim in splendidis officiis jam sunt constituti et titulo Doctorum, Licentiatorumque gaudent; partim vero Practici vivunt famigerabiles." J. H. Gramann from Moscow is listed first on the following list of 22 counsellors. Ibid, D3r. The number of authors of consilia listed in "Mercklin's" bibliography

and support was the genesis of new scientific societies, which encouraged the literary works of their members by for example publishing professional journals to which many physicians contributed their observations.[279]

The progress of the period sped up the process between the compilation of the manuscript and its publication. The shorter amounts of time between those operations confirm the popularity of genres tied to practice. Authors of consilia could thus in greater measure take charge of editorial work and mostly lived to see the final result, which in the publication of consilia or consultations in the 16th century was not at all common (at least for the authors of the selected group of physicians).[280] Naturally, in the 17th century many consilia were published after the deaths of their authors, for example the collections of the consilia of Italian physician M. Malpighi (d. 1694) or of G. H. Welsch (d. 1677), the later publications of the works of Mermann and de Baillou, as well as the numerous reeditions of the consilia of various centuries.

The term "consultatio" began to appear more often in the titles of collections and anthologies written in Latin and published in print in this period. "Consultationes medicae/medicinales" denotes the same professional act as consilia (advice recorded in writing and sent to a distant patient) and at the same time these genres overlap with medical correspondence.[281] The editor of Linden's bibliography, G. A. Mercklin, considered the terms consultatio and consilium synonyms.[282] The already mentioned W. Rolfinck defined the differences between these terms in the chapter "About the Authors of Consilia, Consultations and Observations" in his work in the following manner: "These three titles appear in the works of older as well as current [authors]. Many favor the title "Observations," which are ... for the most

from the year 1686 is not at all enormous, but one must note that this list records exclusively consilia that were printed and the list cannot be complete. Lindenius Renovatus contains 108 names of physicians who wrote consilia or consultations (three of them however lived in the 15th cent.). For more details see Mercklinus, *Lindenius Renovatus*, 35, "Consilia Medica."

279 The first and for Central Europe most important learned society was the Academia Imperialis Leopoldina Naturae Curiosorum (Academia Leopoldina), established in 1652 in Schweinfurt, which brought together exclusively physicians. Doctor E. Gockel, about whom we will speak later, in the introduction to the publication of his consilia, mentions that some had already been published in the scientific journal published by the above-mentioned academy. E.g., Gockelius, *Gallicinium medico-practicum*, 12r. "... aliquot consilia et observationes meas medicas, quae Ephemeridibus Curiosorum jamdudum insertae sunt, hisce praesentibus addere..."

280 As always, this does not apply without exception, J.A. Fischer (d. 1729) edited his cases 16 years later.

281 For more on the significance of consultations in medical correspondence of the 17th century and its typology see Steinke and Stuber, "Medical Correspondence," 139-60.

282 See Mercklinus, *Lindenius Renovatus*, 36. "Consultationes: Vid. Consilia Medica."

part identical to [those] others. Consilia are the results of consultations and those [consultations] precede them. Observations are born of consultations and consilia. "[283]

The designation of "consultation literature" is widely used even in modern studies dealing with the manuscript medical correspondence of the 17th and 18th centuries.[284] These works have provided new information concerning English, French and German consultations and point to some new aspects that deserve closer attention. For example, the studied archival materials indicate that starting in the 17th century, the number of patients from the lower classes started to increase;[285] among consultation clients in France a considerable number of patients from among the ranks of tradespeople were recorded.[286] It also appears that greater attention began to be given to women, who represented an insignificant number among recipients of consilia published in print in the 16th century.[287] Manuscript records have preserved more so-called "request letters" (in French-speaking regions called *mémoires*), which indicate that from the mid-17th century, these requests for consilia began to be written to a greater extent not by attending physicians, but by patients themselves or their relatives, of course not in Latin.[288] However, in collections published in print in Latin these trends are not observable.

283 Rolfinckius, *Ordo ... continens Consilia medica*, Lib. I. Sect. I., 18, Caput X. De scriptoribus consiliorum, consultationum et observationum. „Tres hi tituli occurrunt in monumentis veterum et recentiorum. Observationum inscriptiones placent multis, quae tamen ipsa in re, maxima ex parte cum prioribus conveniunt. Consilia sunt effectus consultationum: hae praevii actus. Observationes emergunt ex consultationibus et consiliis."

284 E.g., Brockliss, "Consultation by Letter," 79-117; Wild, *Medicine-by-Post*; Dinges and Barras, *Krankheit in Briefen*; Weston, *Medical Consulting by Letter*; Dinges et al., Medical Practice, passim.

285 An increase in the numbers of patients from the lower social classes is also observed in the records of actual consultations of physicians of the period. For more on the number of patients and the representation of women among them see Baschin et al., "Doctors and Their Patients," 39-70.

286 Weston, *Medical Consulting*, 44; Stolberg, "Kommunikative Praktiken," 114.

287 Despite this, the number of men evidently continued to exceed that of women. Among the correspondents of renowned surgeon L. Heister men predominated over women by a ratio of 2.2:1. For more see Ruisinger, "Chirurgie im Brief," 133. In collections published in Latin print, there is a markedly greater number of female patients in sections dedicated to headaches. E.g., T. von Güldenklee, *Opera medico-practica*, 1-76, Casuum Medicinalium Liber I. de Affectibus Capitis almost 30% of the consilia were written for women.

288 Weston, *Medical Consulting*, 71; Ruisinger, "Chirurgie im Brief," 136. This of course does not apply without exception. In the consultations of French chemist and physician E. F. Geoffroy (1672-1731) there are often request letters mediated by attending physicians, pharmacists and surgeons who evidently worked as rural physicians Brockliss, "Consultation by Letter," 87. Weston also confirms that surgeons became the most frequent intermediaries for writing "request" letters. For more see Weston, *Medical Consulting*, 44.

The approach to printed publications, their structure and the form of consilia published not only in the 17th but also 18th centuries, did not markedly change in any way. Of course, each editor brought his individual spirit into his work; nevertheless, the editors of the 16th-century collections that were closely examined in detail also did the same. It will evidently surprise no one that authors dedicated their works to their patrons or employers and that the same motives as given by their predecessors in the previous generation appear in the introductions.[289] This motivation was enriched by the publisher of the consilia of the famous M. Malpighi, physician H. Gaspari, who wanted to refute rumors that Malpighi excelled only in theory. However, in 1673, I.F. Thiermair summed up the common motives of his colleagues in the foreword to the publication of his consilia in this way:

> "Many authors ... when they publish their works, excuse these actions in various ways: As the cause, they mention the requests of students, wishes of friends, orders of superiors, longings to please their fellow man, strengthening of the reipublica litteraria ... I admit that no one can disparage these reasons and even I highly praise them ... With the permission of all men of letters, I however tell you [this]: today the main cause of writing is a sort of symptom of a new disease, which has been spreading throughout Europe for about 50 years and is very contagious. It is a sort of creative itch, which pesters the creative spirit of physicians for so long until the itchy matter comes out of the pregnant brain into the light in a sort of birth with the assistance of a midwife, [which is] publication ..."[290]

The social status of patients whose cases were included in Latin printed publications, did not change in any way in either the 17th or 18th century – citizens of the wealthy classes continued to predominate.[291] This is confirmed

289 The words of the editor L. Schröckius: "...non aegrorum tantum particulari commodo, sed et publicae utilitati...," Welschius, *Curationum propriarum*, A2r.; or editor H. Gaspari: "... Auctori gloriae et populi incolumitati, et Reipublicae Literariae utilitati...," Malpighius, *Consultaionum medicinalium centuria*, Bv. – Ba r., can serve as an example. The same goes for the authors, e.g.: Fortis, *Consultationum et responsionum*, 3r. "... a me habitas Consultationes ..., huc illuc transmissas, ac dispersas, Amicorum consilio, atque tandem Patrono imperante, in unum recolligendas curavi, ut, ... in aegrotantium auxilium quisque depromere possit;" Thoner, *Observationum medicinalium libri*, 5v. "... ad procurandam publicam utilitatem;" or Ruff, *Consultationes medicae*, 4v. "... in gratiam maxime juniorum et in stimulum veteranorum."

290 Thiermair, *Scholiorum et Consiliorum*, 2r.

291 Even here there are exceptions, e.g., Fischer, *Consilia medica continuata*, 154, Cons. XXVIII. "Ancilla quaedam conqueritur... [a servant-maid complained];" T. von Güldenklee, *Opera medico-practica*, 90-1, Casus VII. "...piscatoris cuiusdam uxor...[a fisherman's wife]..." etc.

by the titles or the social status of the patients presented by the physician.[292] The stance of physicians towards specifying patients by name differed with each individual. On the one hand, stood the absolute refusal to dishonor noble patients by publicizing their diseases, as expressed by Paduan professor of medicine R. Fortis (d.1676), while on the other stood Ulm physician A. Thoner (d.1655) who mentioned the names and standing of patients very consistently.[293] It is understandable that for example military physician A. Deodatus (d.1676), who served in the camps of the French Army and in city hospitals, mentioned by name only his important patients in his collection of observations, histories and consilia.[294] Like most other physicians, he did so either due to a desire to demonstrate through them his renown as a physician, or because he only remembered these patients by name. If a physician included cases of unimportant persons in his publication, they must have been interesting and unusual cases of diseases or treatments and patients were not usually named. An exception was the physician from Ulm, E. Gockel (d.1703) – if he knew the name, he included it, regardless of whether the person was an aristocrat or a common soldier.[295] It should also be. noted that names of patients appear more frequently in records from the first half of the 17th century and more so in observations, histories or subsequently recorded cases, than in "real" consilia.[296]

The names of physicians involved in the case appear far more often. Editors, usually the same persons as the authors, began to include complete "request letters" in publications, which with exceptions was not common in collections of the 16th century. Although according to archival research, written communication between the physician and patient grew in importance, one can contend that exclusively consilia shared among professionals were put into printed form. Direct communication of the patient (or a relative) with the counsellor was occasionally even included in printed editions of counsellor collections but comprise a very small minority.

292 Fischer, *Consilia medica continuata*, 18, Cons. III. "Civis ex Primariis Urbis ...;" 67, Cons. X. "Mercator ex Comitatu Mansfeldiae...;" 23-4, Cons. IV. "Studiosi Lipsienses ..."

293 Fortis, *Consultationum et responsionum*, 4v. "Aegrotantium nomina addere indecorum semper putavi, siquidem morbosas Religiosorum, Magnatum ac Principum affectiones Mundo palam facere prorsus dedecet." Thoner, *Observationum medicinalium libri*, 73, Obs. XXI. "... Marcus a Lapheim, Praefectus Generos. D. Fuggerorum in Weissenhorn..."

294 Deodatus, *Valetudinarium*, 84. "... Aluysius [sic] Vallaressus Venetus Orator a Legatione sua Anglicana recens, in Castris nostris ..."

295 E. Gockel described for example the case of a thief named Nicolaus Gerber who, thanks to Gockel's successful treatment, did not escape his assessed punishment and could be executed. Gockelius, *Gallicinium medico-practicum*, Centuria I., 132-4, Cons. XXXIV.

296 For more on related genres see chap. 3.2. of this work.

Similar variability is also seen in the inclusion of the dates on which consilia were written. For example, professor of the faculty of medicine in Erfurt J. A. Fischer (d. 1729) mentioned dates and locations very meticulously, so we know that all cases recorded in his publication from the year 1706 occurred between May 1690 and November 1691.[297] J. A. Fischer divided his consilia into two parts: the first including the date and location of the event, recorded the story of the patient and "anamnesis," or the "request letter" of a colleague. In the second part, the "Responsio," he described his treatment procedure, diagnosis and prescription, and the date often appears even here. In written responses to "request letters," so in real consilia, the date is provided consistently. And on the contrary: in the collections of consilia, consultations or observations of the physicians M. Malpighi, R. I. Fortis, F. I. Thiermair or A. Thoner, the date information does not appear at all, and in the collections of A. Deodatus, E. Gockel, B. T. Güldenklee (d. 1667) and others irregularly. Essentially the same applies to the specification of the location of writing, which could be an important lead for estimating the reach of the renown of a counsellor, or the speed of postal transportation. Publishing these details was the responsibility of the editor and certainly had an influence on whether the editor was the author himself.

The points to which attention was paid in researching selected publications of the 16th century included the number of consilia in collections and anthologies. The number of consilia in randomly screened works from the following century range from just seven consilia of Savon physician A. Gigard to several hundred in the collections of J. A. Welsch, or E. Gockel.[298] The number of consilia is often already mentioned in the title of the book, nevertheless rarely does this actually correspond.[299] Obtaining more precise information is made more difficult by the variability of the utilized genres. For example, the physician F.I. Thiermair did not number individual consilia, but only chapters (capita), which could include the request letter, several consilia, an analysis (scholion) and sometimes even a treatise about the discussed disease;[300] A. Gigard enhanced his consilia with observations, scholion, and "questions";[301] and military physician A. Deodatus completely left out numbering and freely

297 Fischer, *Consilia medica continutata.*

298 Gigard, *Consilia medica.*

299 Welschius, *Curationum exotericarum chiliades II. et Consiliorum ... centuriae quatuor*; Welschius, *Curationum ... Decades X.*; Gockelius, *Observationum ... centuriae duae*; Malpighius, *Consultationum ... centuria*; Fortis, *Consultationum ... centuriae quatuor,* etc.

300 Thiermair, *Scholiorum et Consiliorum*, e.g. Lib. I., 181-96, Cap. XV.; Lib. II., 42-64, Cap. III.

301 Gigard, *Consilia medica*, 65-74, Observatio rara; 89-95 Scholia; pg. 95-9 Quaestio celeberrima; 129-35 Scholia. For function of "scholion" see also Calabritto, "Curing Melancholy," 629.

ordered consilia, request letters, his own and others' observations, histories, or memoirs of his professors. The published works cannot be called collections of consilia and for the most part one physician cannot be designated as the author.[302] Regardless of whether they were published under the name consilia, consultations, casus, historiae, or observations – all related forms, to which a separate sub-section will be devoted, intermingle in the publications.

A novelty in prints of the 17th and 18th centuries was illustrations, which were not used in the consilia collections and anthologies of the 16th century, or at least until now have not been discovered in any of the studied consilia publications. Drawings depict the injuries or disabilities of a patient, but unfortunately one cannot in most cases determine whether the drawing was sent by the distant person requesting the consilium, or the counsellor sketched it himself in the course of an actual consultation.[303] The editor included astrological drawings in Welsch's collections published after his death.[304] Although illustrations are not at all frequent in printed publications of this type, one can perceive these pictures as an expression of the growing effort to illustrate on the part of physicians and the improving technical possibilities that the 17th and 18th centuries brought.

The language question is also worth paying attention to. Already in the 16th century, consilia or appendices in vernacular languages appeared in consultation publications. Usually, however, the consilia were translated into the international language of Latin to reach the widest possible readership among scholars. W. Wild states that in eighteenth-century British consultation letters and literature, English predominated in communication and Latin was used only in consultation with foreign physicians.[305] R. Weston came to a similar conclusion regarding the consultations in France and added that the part of the consultations or letters of request written in Latin had been translated into French for the press.[306] The trend to incorporate vernacular notes into Latin prints grew in the collections and anthologies of physicians, whose native language was German as well. In the introduction to his work from the year 1662, B. T. von Güldenklee mentioned: "what was written in German, I have left in German. Not that it would have been difficult to translate into Latin, but it is of no use."[307] The question of when

302 Exceptions are the collections of M. Malpighi, or R.I. Fortis.

303 Fischer, *Consilia medica continuata*, 242, 265; Thiermair, *Scholiorum et consiliorum*, 121, 196.

304 Welschius, *Curationum propriarum*, 11, 38, 54, 72 and many others, without pagination.

305 Wild, *Consulting-by-Post*, 20.

306 Weston, *Medical Consulting*, 28.

307 T. von Güldenklee, *Opera medico-practica*, 445. "Germanice scripta, Germanice inserui; Non quod latinitate donare arduum foret, sed quia supervacaneum."

and under what circumstances vernacular languages prevailed not only in communication, but also in consortium editions would certainly be worth closer attention in the future.

In conclusion, just a small comment regarding the content of consilia. The 17th and 18th centuries witnessed (in addition to wars) important technical and scientific discoveries, so in particular the 17th century is sometimes called the century of the Scientific Revolution. However, medical discoveries did not have a stronger influence on the content and treatment procedures recorded in consilia and consultations. R.I. Fortis clearly expressed the general opinion in the preface to the publication of his consultations: "... know that I wrote some of them [consultations] before I agreed with circulation of the blood. The main proof that the truth remains hidden for me was ... the dispute of many professors of anatomy ..., so because I was never very interested in those things about which I knew that to professional learning and methodological practice ... add, take away, [or about them] change nothing at all."[308]

The above-outlined characterization of consultation records of the 17th and 18th centuries is not exhaustive. However, we have hopefully succeeded at least in outline in demonstrating that the development of consilia literature did not in the course of the centuries undergo any revolutionary transformation or significant watershed event that would radically change the form, structure, or their purpose. Nevertheless, it can be considered that there has been a certain shift in the consuls of this period, which is likely to have manifested itself in all the scientific literature. It is primarily an extension of the desire for the literary self-presentation of doctors, which was highlighted by F. Thiermair. His colleague Timaeus also confirmed the large increase in medical literature production with his concern about whether future generations would have anything to write about at all.[309] If Mr. Thiermair's time estimate is correct and this "disease" began to spread around the 1520s, it may be evidence of the increasing importance of individuals to actively engage in "Respublica medica," the emphasis that doctors placed on current practical medicine, and perhaps the now debatable "scientific revolution of the 17th century." However, these are only assumptions; guaranteed conclusions would require much more thorough and broader study and a better analysis of all external and internal aspects. Some of these will be mentioned in the following overview section.

308 Fortis, *Consultationum et responsionum*, 4v.

309 T. von Güldenklee, *Opera medico-practica*, Ir. "...seculi huius est felicitas, in quo in tantum literarum studia evecta sunt fastigium, ut nihil fere reliquum esse videatur, in quo futurorum occupari possit seculorum diligentia."

Bibliography

Abe, Horst R. *Die Erfurter medizinische Fakultät in den Jahren 1392-1524*. Beiträge zur Geschichte der Universität Erfurt, 17, Leipzig: J.A. Barth, 1974.

Agrimi, Jole and Crisciani, Chiara. *Les consilia medicaux*. Trans. Caroline Viola. Turnhout: Brepols, 1994.

Almási, Gábor. *The Uses of Humanism. Johannes Sambucus (1531-1584), Andreas Dudith (1533-1589), and the Republic of Letters in East Central Europe.* Leiden: Brill, 2009.

Archivio di Stato, Firenze, Fondo Ducato di Urbino, CL. I, F. 218, fol. 131r.-166v.

Arrizabalaga, Jon, Montserrat Cabré, Luis Cifuentes, and Fernando Salmón, eds. *Galen and Galenism. Theory and Medical Practice from Antiquity to the European Renaissance*, Farnham: Ashgate Press, 2002.

Baader, Gerhard. "Anatomie, Konsilienliteratur und der neue Naturalismus in Italien im Spätmittelalter und Frühumanismus." In *Die Kunst und das Studium der Natur vom 14. zum 16. Jahrhundert*, edited by Wolfram Prinz, Andreas Beyer, and Gerhard Baader, 127-41. Cologne: Weinheim VCH, 1987.

Baader, Gerhard. "Medizinisches Reformdenken und Arabismus im Deutschland des 16. Jahrhunderts," *Sudhoffs Archiv* 63, no. 3 (1979): 261-96.

Ballonius, Guillielmus [sic]. *Consiliorum medicinalium liber tertius et postremus, item paradigmata et historiae morborum ob raritatem observatione dignissimae.* Paris: Iacob Quesnel, 1649.

Ballonius, Gulielmus. *Consiliorum medicinalium liber primus.* Paris: Iacob Quesnel, 1635.

Ballonius, Gulielmus. *Consiliorum medicinalium liber secundus.* Paris: Iacob Quesnel, 1636.

Baschin, Marion, Elisabeth Dietrich-Daum, and Iris Ritzmann. "Doctors and Their Patients in the Seventeenth to Nineteenth Centuries." In *Medical Practice, 1600-1900. Physicians and Their Patients, edited by* Martin Dinges, Kay Peter Jankrift, Sabine Schlegemilch, and Michael Stolberg, 39-70. *Leiden: Brill-Rodopi, 2016.*

Baumann, Werner. "Ernst Friedrich von Baden-Durlach, Felix Platter und Poland." *Theologische Zeitschrift* 59, no. 4 (2003): 335-41.

Baumann, Werner. *Ernst Friedrich von Baden-Durlach. Die Bedeutung der Religion für Leben und Politik eines süddeutschen Fürsten im Zeitalter der Gegenreformation.* Stuttgart: W. Kohlhammer, 1962.

Biblioteca Oliveriana, Pesaro, MS 429/31, fol. 163r., 164r.

Binz, C. "Wier, Johann." *Allgemeine Deutsche Biographie,* 42 (1897): 266-70. https://www.deutsche-biographie.de/pnd118632043.html#adbcontent (13.5.2021)

Brockliss, Laurence. "Consultation by Letter in Early Eighteenth-Century Paris: The Medical Practice of Etienne-Francois Geoffroy," In *French Medical Culture in the Nineteenth Century*, edited by Ann la Berge, and Mordechai Feingold, 79-117. Amsterdam: Editions Rodopi, 1994.

Brodman, Estelle. *The Development of Medical Bibliography.* Baltimore: Medical Library Association, 1954.

Buršíková, Bohdana. "Sbírka konsilií císařského lékaře Christophora Guarinoniho" [The Consilia Collection of Imperial Physician Christophoro Guarinoni], *Dějiny věd a techniky* [*History of Sciences and Technology*] 34, no. 1 (2001): 23-38.

Bylebyl, Jerome J. "The School of Padua: Humanistic Medicine in the Sixteenth Century." In *Health, Medicine, and Mortality in the Sixteenth Century*, edited by Charles Webster, 335-70. Cambridge: Cambridge University Press, 1979.

Calabritto, Monica. "Curing Melancholia in Sixteenth-Century Medical Consilia between Theory and Practice," *Medicina nei Secoli* (*Journal of the History of Medicine*) 24, no. 3 (2012): 627-64.

Calabritto, Monica. "*Medicina practica*, Consilia and the Illnesses of the Head in Girolamo Mercuriale and Giulio Cesare Claudini. Similarities and Differences of the Sexes," *Medicina e Storia* 13, no. 4 (2006): 63-83.

Capivaccius, Hieronymus. *Opera omnia ... qua editione, tum Capivaccii plurima typis hactenus novum vulgata in lucem proferuntur: tum depravatissimi Gallorum atque Italorum codices penitus abolentur...* Frankfurt am Main: Paltheniana, 1603.

Černý, Karel. *Mor 1480-1730. Epidemie v lékařských traktátech raného novověku* [*The Plague 1480-1730. Epidemics in Early Modern Medical Treatises*]. Prague: Karolinum, 2014.

Cohn, Ferdinand. "Scholz von Rosenau, Laurentius." *Allgemeine Deutsche Biographie,* 32 (1891): 229-30. https://www.deutsche-biographie.de/pnd116911670.html#adbcontent (1.4.2021)

Consilia diversorum Medicorum circa nervorum debilitatem Ill. D.D. Guilhelmi a S. Clemente etc., sign. D. D. II. 22, Strahovská knihovna Kláštera premonstrátů [Strahov Library of the Strahov Premonstratensians Monastery], Prague.

Cornarius, Diomedes. *Consiliorum medicinalium habitorum in consultationibus a clarissimis atque expertissimis, apud diversos aegrotos, partim defunctis, partim adhuc superstitibus medicis, tractatus.* Leipzig: Michaël Lantzenberger, 1599.

Crato a Kraftheim, Ioannes. *Consiliorum et epistolarum medicinalium liber, ex collectaneis ... Petri Monavii ... selectus ... nunc primum a Laurentio Scholzio ... editus.* Frankfurt am Main: Andreae Wecheli heredes, 1591.

Crato a Kraftheim, Ioannes. *Consiliorum et epistolarum medicinalium Ioh. Cratonis ..., liber secundus; nunc primum studio ... Laurentii Scholzii ... editus.* Frankfurt am Main: Andreae Wecheli heredes, 1592.

Crato a Kraftheim, Ioannes. *Consiliorum et epistolarum medicinalium Ioh. Cratonis ..., liber quartus; nunc primum studio ... Laurentii Scholzii ... editus.* Frankfurt am Main: Andreae Wecheli heredes, 1593.

Crato a Kraftheim, Ioannes. *Consiliorum et epistolarum medicinalium Ioh. Cratonis ..., liber quintus; nunc primum labore ... Laurentii Scholzii ... in lucem editus.* Frankfurt am Main: Andreae Wecheli heredes, 1594.

Crato a Kraftheim, Ioannes. *Consiliorum et epistolarum medicinalium Io. Cratonis ..., liber sextus; nunc primum studio ... Laurentii Scholzii ... editus.* Hanau: haeredes Ioannis Aubrii, 1611.

Crato a Kraftheim, Ioannes. *Consiliorum et epistolarum medicinalium Io. Cratonis ... liber septimus; nunc primum labore ... Laurentii Scholzii ... editus.* Hanau: haeredes Ioannis Aubrii, 1611.

Crato a Kraftheim, Ioannes. *Consiliorum et epistolarum medicinalium Ioh. Cratonis ... liber tertius; nunc primum labore ... Laurentii Scholzii ... editus.* Frankfurt am Main: Andreae Wecheli heredes, 1592.

Crisciani, Chiara. "Consilia, responsi, consulti. I pareri del medico tra insegnamento e professione." In *Consilium. Teorie e pratiche del consigliare nella cultura medievale*, edited by Carla Casagrande, Chiara Crisciani, and Silvana Vecchio, 259-79. Firenze: Sismel, 2004.

Crisciani, Ciara. "'Exempla in medicina'. Epistemologia, insegnamento, retorica (Secoli XIII-XV). Una proposta di ricerca." In *Exempla medicorum. Die Ärzte und ihre Beispiele (14.-18. Jahrhundert)*, edited by Mariacarla Gadebusch Bondio, and Thomas Ricklin, 89-108. Firenze: Sismel, 2008.

Deer Richardson, Linda. "The Generation of Disease: Occult Causes and Diseases of the Total Substance." In *The Renaissance of the Sixteenth Century,* edited by Andrew Wear, Roger French, and Iain Lonie, 175-94. Cambridge: Cambridge University Press, 1985.

Deodatus, Alexandrus. *Valetudinarium, seu Observationum, curationum, et consiliorum medicinalium satura.* Leiden: Johan. Elzevier, 1660.

Dieckhöfer, Klemens. "Solenander, Reiner." *Neue Deutsche Biographie*, 24 (2010): 549. https://www.deutsche-biographie.de/pnd124555322.html#ndbcontent (2.6.2021)

Dinges, Martin, and Vincent Barras, eds. *Krankheit in Briefen im deutschen und französischen Sprachraum 17.-21. Jahrhundert.* Stuttgart: Franz Steiner Verlag, 2007.

Dinges, Martin, *Kay Peter Jankrift, Sabine Schlegemilch, and Michael Stolberg, eds. Medical Practice, 1600-1900. Physicians and Their Patients. Trans. Margot Saar. Leiden: Brill, 2016.*

Divišová, Bohdana. "Ärzte mit den Nachnamen Guarinoni – Alle die Kaiserlichen Guarinoni," *Studia Rudolphina* 11 (2011): 89-101.

Eis, Gerhard. Crato von Craffthein, Johannes." *Neue Deutsche Biographie*, 3 (1957): 402-3. https://www.deutsche-biographie.de/pnd119440067.html#ndbcontent (3.5.2021)

Evans, Robert J.W. *Rudolf II and His World: a Study in Intellectual History 1576-1612.* Oxford: Clarendon Press, 1984.

Fernelius, Ioannes. *Consiliorum medicinalium liber quadringentarum consultationum selectus.* Turin: Gio. Dominicus Tarinus, 1589.

Fernelius, Ioannes. *Consiliorum medicinalium liber, cui accesserunt responsa ...* Leiden: Thomas Soubron et Moysen de Prez, 1597.

Fernellius, Ioannes. *Consiliorum liber* [sic], *cui accesserunt responsa ... medicorum Parisiensium.* Paris: Aegidius Beysius, 1585.

Fernellius, Ioannes. *Consiliorum medicinalium liber. Ex eius adversariis quadringentarum consultationum selectus.* Paris: Aegidius Beysius, 1582.

Fischer, Johann Andreas. *Consilia medica continuata.* Frankfurt am Main: Joh. Maximil. a Sande, 1706.

Forrester, John M., and John Henry, *Jean Fernel's On the Hidden Causes of Things: Form, Souls, and Occult Diseases in Renaissance Medicine.* Leiden: Brill 2004.

Fortis, Raymundus Ioannes. *Consultationum et responsionum medicinalium centuriae quatuor. Accesserunt eiusdem consilia ...* Genova: Sumptibus Leonardi Chovët, 1677.

Fortuna di, Stefania. "Trincavelli, Vittore." *Dizionario Biografico degli Italiani*, 96, 2019. https://www.treccani.it/enciclopedia/vittore-trincavelli_(Dizionario-Biografico) (12.3.2020)

French, Roger. *Canonical Medicine. Gentile da Foligno and Scholasticism.* Leiden: Brill, 2001.

Frühneuzeitliche Ärztebriefe des deutschsprachigen Raums (1500-1700), www.aerztebriefe.de [12.1.2021].

Fuchs, Franz. "Schedel, Hartmann." *Neue Deutsche Biographie*, 22 (2005): 600-2. https://www.deutsche-biographie.de/pnd118754211.html#ndbcontent (11.11.2020)

Gallus, Paschalis. *Bibliotheca medica. Sive catalogus illorum, qui ex professo artem medicam in hunc usque annum scriptis illustraruntur.* Basel: Conrad Waldkirch, 1590.

García-Ballester, Luis. "Galen as a Clinician: II. Diagnosis and prognosis." In *Galen and Galenism. Theory and Medical Practice from Antiquity to the European Renaissance*, editedy by Jon Arrizabalaga, Montserrat Cabré, Luis Cifuentes, and Fernando Salmón, 1640-2. Farnham: Ashgate Press, 2002.

García-Ballester, Luis. "On the Origin of the 'six non-natural things' in Galen," *Sudhoffs Archiv für Geschichte der Medizin. Beiheft* 32 (1993): 105-15.

Gerabek, Werner. "Thiermair, Franz Ignaz." *Neue Deutsche Biographie*, 26, (2016): 133. https://www.deutsche-biographie.de/pnd118040065.html#ndbcontent

Gigard, Antonius. *Consilia medica fere consultatoria methodo digesta, circa varias, maxima parte implicatas, quasdam raro insurgentes, tamen experimento compertas, ... aegritudines.* Mondovi: Franciscus Maria Gisland, 1666.

Gliozzi di, Giuliano. "Capodivacca, Girolamo," in: *Dizionario Biografico degli Italiani*, 18, 1975. https://www.treccani.it/enciclopedia/girolamo-capodivacca_(Dizionario-Biografico) (8.3.2020)

Gockelius, Eberhardus. *Gallicinium medico-practicum, sive Consiliorum, observationum et curationum medicinalium centuriae duae cum dimidia*, Ulm: Georgius Wilhelmus Kühnen, 1700.

Guarinonius, Christophorus. *Consilia medicinalia, in quibus universa praxis medica exacte pertractatur.* Venice: Thoma Baglioni, 1610.

Güldenklee, Baldassar Timaeus von. *Opera medico-practica.* Leipzig: impensis Ch. Kirchneri, 1677.

Gunnoe Jr., Charles D., and Jole Shackelford. "Johannes Crato von Krafftheim (1519-1585): Imperial Physician, Irenicist, and Anti-Paracelsian." In *Ideas and Cultural Margins in Early Modern Germany*, edited by Elisabeth Plummer, and Robin B. Barnes, 201-16. Farnham: Ashgate Press, 2009.

Hankinson, Jim R. "Philosophy of Nature." In *The Cambridge Companion to Galen*, edited by Jim R. Hankinson, 210-41. Cambridge: Cambridge University Press, 2008.

Hausenblásová, Jaroslava, and Michal Šroněk. *Urbs Aurea: Prague of Emperor Rudolf II.* Prag: Gallery, 1997.

Hirsch, August, "Cornarius, Janus." *Allgemeine Deutsche Biographie* 4, (1876): 481. https://www.deutsche-biographie.de/pnd11769875X.html#adbcontent (15.12.2020)

Hirsch, August. *Biographisches Lexikon der hervorragenden Ärzte aller Zeiten und Völker*, 6. Wien: Urban und Schwarzenberg, 1888.

Hirsch, August. *Biographisches Lexikon der hervorragenden Ärzte aller Zeiten und Völker*, 2, Wien-Leipzig: Urban und Schwarzenberg, 1885.

Hlaváčková, Ludmila, and Petr Svobodný. *Dějiny lékařství v českých zemích* [*The History of Medicine in the Bohemian Crown Lands*] Prague: Triton, 2004.

Hlaváčková, Ludmila, Petr Svobodný, Karel Beránek, Jana Nosáková, and Eva Rozsívalová. *Biografický slovník pražské lékařské fakulty 1348-1939* [*The Biographical Dictionary of the Prague Faculty of Medicine 1348-1939*]. 2, Prague: Univerzita Karlova, 1993.

Jacquart, Danielle. "Medical Practice in Paris in the First Half of the Fourteenth Century." In *Practical Medicine from Salerno to the Black Death*, edited by Luis G. Ballester, Roger French, Jon Arrizabalaga, and Andrew Cunningham, 186-210. Cambridge: Cambridge University Press, 1994.

Keil, Gundolf. "Konsilium." In *Lexikon des Mittelalters*, edited by Robert H. Bautier, and Robert Auty, 5, 1370-1. Munich: Artemis, 1991.

Klestinec, Cynthia. "Medical Education in Padua: Students, Faculty and Facilities." In *Centres of Medical Excellence? Medical Travel and Education in Europe, 1500-1789*, edited by Ole P. Grell, Andrew Cunningham, and Jon Arrizabalaga, 193-220. Farnham: Ashgate Press, 2010.

l.u. "Wittich, Johannes," *Allgemeine Deutsche Biographie*, 43, 1898, 635. https://www.deutsche-biographie.de/pnd118880578.html#adbcontent (8.11.2020)

Lindenius, Ioannes Antonides. *De scriptis medicis libri duo.* Amsterdam: Iohannes Blaev, 1637.

Lockwood, Dean P. "A Medieval Consilium: Ugo Benzi (1376-1439)." In *Health, Disease and Society in Europe 1500-1800. A Source Book,* edited by Peter Elmer, and Ole P. Grell, 5-8. Manchester: Manchester University Press, 2004.

Lonie, Iain M. "The Paris Hippocratics: Teaching and Research in Paris in the Second Half of the Sixteenth Century." In *The Renaissance of the Sixteenth Century,* edited by Andrew Wear, Roger French, and Iain Lonie, 155-74. Cambridge: Cambridge University Press, 1985.

Maclean, Ian. *Learning and the Market Place. Essays in the History of the Early Modern Book.* Leiden: Brill, 2009.

Maclean, Ian. *Logic, Signs and Nature in the Renaissance. The Case of Learned Medicine.* Cambridge: Cambridge University Press, 2002.

Maclean, Ian. *Scholarship, Commerce, Religion: the Learned Book in the Age of Confessions, 1560-1630.* Cambridge (MA): Harvard University Press, 2012.

Malpighius, Marcellus. *Consultationum medicinalium centuria prima.* Padua: Typographia Seminarii, 1713.

Matthaeus, Ioannes. *Consilia medica diversorum auctorum, pro Ill. Principe ... Ernesto Friderico, Marchione Badense.* Franfkurt am Mein: Collegium Musarum Palthenianum, 1608.

Mercklinus, Georgius Abrahamus. *Lindenius Renovatus, sive de scriptis medicis libri duo.* Nuremberg: 1686.

Mercklinus, Georgius Abrahamus. *Cynosura medica, sive de scriptis medicis liber II.* Nuremberg: 1686.

Mermannus, Thomas. *Consultationes ac responsiones medicae, ... opera et studio Francisci ... Thiermairii,... Ex variis manu-scriptis hinc inde sparsis, ... conquisitae: partim ex Germanico et Italico idiomate in Latinum versae, partim ..., annotationibus et remediis succedaneis, auctae.* Ingolstadt: Joannes Phillippus Zinck, 1675.

Meuthen, Erich. *Kölner Universitäts Geschichte. Die alte Universität.* Cologne: Böhlau Verlag, 1988.

Montanus, Ioannes Baptista. *Consultationum medicarum opus absolutissimum. In quo ad consilia omnia prius edita, ... accesserunt centum fere nunquam antea typis expressa ... opera Ioannis Cratonis.* Basel: Petri, 1565.

Muccillo di, Maria. "Da Monte, Giovanni," *Dizionario Biografico degli Italiani,* 32 (1986). https://www.treccani.it/enciclopedia/da-monte-giovanni-battista-detto-montano_(Dizionario-Biografico) [4.3.2020]

Oszczanowski, Piotr. "Wroclawski ogród Laurentiusa Scholtze st. (1552-1599) – sceneria spotkań elity intelektualnej końca XVI. Wieku" [The Wroclaw Garden of Lorenz Scholz – The Backdrop for Meetings of the Intellectual Elite of the End of the 16th Century]. In *Ślaska republika uczonych – Schlesische Gelehrtenrepublik*

– *Slezská vědecká obec*, edited by Marek Halub, and Anna Mańko-Matysiak, 99-125. Wroclaw: Neisse-Verlag, 2004.

Palmer, Richard. "Girolamo Mercuriale and the Plague of Venice." In *Girolamo Mercuriale. Medicina e cultura nell'Europa del cinquecento*, edited by Alessandro Arcangeli, and Vivian Nutton, 51-65. Firenze: L.S. Olschki, 2008.

Pomata, Gianna. "Praxis Historialis: The Uses of Historia in Early Modern Medicine." In *Empiricism and Erudition in Early Modern Europe*, edited by Gianna Pomata, and Nancy G. Siraisi, 105-46. Cambridge (MA)-London: MIT Press 2005.

Prachaticz de, Christianus. *De sanguinis minucione. O pouštění krve*. Ed. and trans. Hana Florianová. Prague: OIKOYMENH 1999.

Quaranta, Alessandra, "Exile Experiences 'Religionis causa' and the Trasmission of Medical Knowledge between Italy and German-Speaking Territories in the Second Half of the Sixteenth Century." In *Fruits of Migration. Heterodox Italian Migrants and Central European Culture 1550-1620*, edited by Cornel Zwierlein, and Vincenzo Lavenia, 72-101. Leiden: Brill, 2018.

Rankin, Alisha. *Panaceia's Doughters: Noblewomen as Healers in Early Modern Germany*. Chicago: The University of Chicago Press, 2013.

Ridder-Symoens de, Hilde. "The Mobility of Medical Students from the Fifteenth to the Eighteenth Centuries: The Institutional Context." In *Centres of Medical Excellence? Medical Travel and Education in Europe, 1500-1789*, edited by Ole P. Grell, Andrew Cunningham, and Jon Arrizabalaga, 47-89. Farnham: Ashgate Press, 2010.

Riha, Ortrun. *Meister Alexanders Monatsregeln: Untersuchungen zu einem spätmittelalterlichen Regimen duodecim mensium mit kritischer Textausgabe*. Pattensen: Horst Wellm, 1985.

Riha, Ortrun. *Wissenorganisation in medizinischen Sammelhandschriften. Klassifikationskriterien und Kombinationsprinzipien bei Texten ohne Werkcharakter.* Wiesbaden: L. Reichert, 1992.

Říhová, Milada. "Regimen sanitatis pro krále Václava" [The Regimen Sanitatis for King Wenceslaus], *Acta Universitatis Carolinae-Historia Universitatis Carolinae Pragensis*, 35, no. 2 (1995): 13-28.

Říhová, Milada. "Středověká pražská regimina" [Medieval Prague Regimina], *Sborník lékařský* [*The Medical Anthology*,] 98, no. 1 (1997): 39-43.

Říhová, Milada. *Dvorní lékař posledních Lucemburků. Albík z Uničova, lékař králů Václava IV. a Zikmunda, profesor pražské univerzity a krátký čas i arcibiskup pražský* [*The Court Physician of the Last Luxembourgs. Albicus of Uniczow, Physician to Kings Wenceslaus IV. and Sigismund, Professor of the University of Prague and Archbishop of Prague for a Short Time*]. Prague: Karolinum, 1999.

Rolfincius, Guernerus. *Ordo et methodus medicinae specialis consultatoriae continens consilia medica ad normam veterum et novorum dogmatum adornata*. Jena: Samuel Krebs, 1669.

Ruff, Ioannes Casparus. *Consultationes Medicae sive Commercium Literarum.* Augsburg: 1777.

Ruisinger, Marion M. "Chirurgie im Brief. Das Beispiel de Konsiliarkorrespondenz Lorenz Heisters (1683-1758)." In *Krankheit in Briefen im deutschen und französischen Sprachraum 17.-21. Jahrhundert*, edited by Martin Dinges, and Vincent Barras, 131-42. Stuttgart: Franz Steiner Verlag, 2007.

Salloch, Sabine. *Das hessische Medizinalwesen unter den Landgrafen Wilhelm IV. und Moritz dem Gelehrten. Rolle und Wirken der fürstlichen Leibärzte*. Ph.D. diss., Marburg, 2006. http://archiv.ub.uni-marburg.de/diss/z2006/0697/pdf/dss.pdf (12.4.2014)

Schenckius, Ioannes Georgius. *Biblia iatrica sive bibliotheca medica macta, continuata.* Frankfurt am Mein: Ioannes Spiess, 1609.

Schipperges, Heinrich. "Regiment der Gesundheit," *Bild der Wissenschaft. Zeitschrift für Naturwissenschaft und Technik in unserer Zeit,* no. 9 (1972): 1309-15.

Scholzius, Laurentius. *Consiliorum medicinalium, conscriptorum a ... exercitatissimis nostrorum temporum medicis liber singularis.* Frankfurt am Mein: Andreae Wecheli Haeredes, 1598.

Schuba, Ludwig. "Die medizinische Fakultät im 15. Jahrhundert." In *Sechshundertjahre Ruprecht-Karls-Universität Heidelberg 1386-1986. Mittelalter und frühe Neuzeit 1386-1803*, edited by Eike Wolgast, 162-87. Heidelberg: Braus 1985.

Sherrington, Charles. *The Endeavour of Jean Fernel.* Cambridge: Cambridge University Press, 1946.

Siraisi, Nancy G. "Avicenna and the Teaching of Practical Medicine." In *Medicine and the Italian Universities, 1250-1600*, edited by Nancy G. Siraisi, 63-78. Leiden: Brill, 2001.

Siraisi, Nancy G. "Giovanni Argenterio: Medical Innovation, Princely Patronage, and Academic Controversy." In *Medicine and the Italian Universities 1250-1600*, edited by Nancy G. Siraisi, 328-55. Leiden: Brill 2001.

Siraisi, Nancy G. "Two Models of Medical Culture, Pietro d'Abano and Taddeo Alderotti." In *Medicine and the Italian Universities 1250-1600*, edited by Nancy G. Siraisi, 77-99. Leiden: Brill 2001.

Siraisi, Nancy G. *Avicenna in Renaissance Italy. The Canon and Medical Teaching in Italian Universities after 1500*. Princeton: Princeton University Press, 1987.

Siraisi, Nancy G. *Communities of Learned Experience. Epistolary Medicine in the Renaissance.* Baltimore: John Hopkins University Press, 2013.

Siraisi, Nancy G. *Medieval and Early Renaissance Medicine. An Introduction to Knowledge and Practice*. Chicago: Chicago University Press, 1990.

Siraisi, Nancy G. *Taddeo Alderotti and His Puppils. Two Generations of Italian Medical Learning*. Princeton: Princeton University Press 1981.

Smolka, Josef. "Hájkův přítel a korespondent Andreas Dudith (1533-1589)" [Hajek's Friend and Correspondent, Andreas Dudith (1533-1589),]. In *Tadeáš Hájek z Hájku,* edited by Pavel Drábek, 125-68. Prague: Práce z dějin techniky a přírodních věd, 2000.

Solenander, Reinerus. *Consiliorum medicinalium sectiones quinque.* Frankfurt am Mein: Andreae Wecheli heredes, 1596.

Spachius, Israel. *Nomenclator scriptorum medicorum.* Frankfurt am Mein: Martin Lechler, 1591.

Stehlíková, Dana. *Od anděliky po zimostráz. Latinský Herbář Křišťana z Prachatic a počátky staročeských herbářů.* [*From Angelica to Boxwood. Latin Herbarium of Křišťan from Prachatice and the Beginnings of Old Bohemian Herbariums*]. Havlíčkův Brod: CDK, 2017.

Steinke, Hubert, and Martin Stuber. "Medical Correspondence in Early Modern Europe. An Introduction," *Gesnerus: Swiss Journal of the History of Medicine and Sciences* 61 (2004): 139-60.

Stolberg, Michael. "Kommunikative Praktiken. Ärztliche Wissensvermittlung am Krankenbett im 16. Jahrhundert." In *Praktiken der frühen Neuzeit. Akteure-Handlungen-Artefakte,* edited by Arndt Brendecke, 111-20. Cologne: Böhlau Verlag, 2015.

Svobodný, Petr. "Lékařská fakulta" [*The Faculty of medicine*] In *Dějiny Univerzity Karlovy I.* [*The History of Charles University*], edited by Michal Svatoš, 183-202. Prague, 1995.

Thiermair, Franciscus Ignatius. *Scholiorum et consiliorum medicorum libri duo.* Munich: Joannes Facklin, 1673

Thoner, Augustinus. *Observationum medicinalium, ... libri quatuor, ... Consultationum ... et Epistolarum Libri Duo.* Ulm: Johannes Gerlin, 1649

Thorndike, Lynn. "'Consilia' and More Works in Manuscripts by G. da Foligno," *Medical History* 3, no. 1 (1959): 8-19.

Thorndike, Lynn. "The Debate for Precedence between Medicine and Law," *Romanic Review* 27 (1936): 185-90.

Trincavellius, Victor. *Consilia medica post editionem Venetam et Lugdunensem, accessione CXXVIII consiliorum locupletata ... Epistolae item... Accessere Tractatus tres ...* Basel: Conradus Valdkirchius, 1587.

Trincavellius, Victor. *Consiliorum medicinalium libri tres; Epistolarum medicinalium libri tres.* Venice: Camillus Borgominerius, 1586.

Uiblein, Paul. "Beziehungen der Wiener Medizin zur Universität Padua im Mittelalter. Mit einem Konsilium des Stadtarztes von Udine Jeremias de Simeonibus für Herzog Albrecht VI. von Österreich." In *Die Universität Wien im Mittelalter: Beiträge und Forschungen,* edited by Paul Uiblein, 143-78. Wien: Universitäts Verlag, 1999.

Venustus, Antonius Maria. *Consilia medica, ... in quibus ... consultandi methodus proponitur, multi morbi ... considerantur.* Venice: Franciscus Zilettus, 1571.

Vermeer, Hans. "Johann Lochners 'Reisekonsilia'," *Sudhoffs Archiv* 56, no. 2 (1972): 145-96.

Victorius, Benedictus. *Medicinalia consilia, ad varia morborum genera ... nunc primum in lucem edita.* Venice: apud Vincentium Valgrisium, 1551.

Victorius, Benedictus. *Medicinalia consilia, ad varia morborum genera.* Venice: Iordan Zillettus, 1556.

Wear, Andrew. "Explorations in renaissance writings on the practice of medicine." In *The Renaissance of the Sixteenth Century,* edited by Andrew Wear, Roger French, and Iain Lonie, 118-45. Cambridge: Cambridge University Press, 1985.

Welschius, Georgius Hieronimus. *Curationum exotericarum chiliades II. et Consiliorum medicinalium centuriae quatuor.* Ulm: Schott, 1676.

Welschius, Georgius Hieronimus. *Curationum propriarum, et Consiliorum medicorum decades X* (opus posthumum). Augsburg: L. Kronegerus et Haeredes Th. Goebelii, 1698.

Weston, Robert. *Medical Consulting by Letter in France, 1665-1789.* Farnham: Ashgate Press, 2013.

Wild, Wayne. *Medicine-by-Post: the Changing Voice of Illness in Eighteenth-Century Britisch Consultation Letters and Literature.* Amsterdam: Rodopi, 2006.

Wittichius, Iohannes. *Nobiliss[imo]rum ... Germaniae Medicorum consilia, observationes atque epistolae medicae.* Leipzig: Henning Grossius, 1604.

www.aerztebriefe.de (Frühneuzeitliche Ärztebriefe des deutschprachigen Raums (1500-1700).

3 Consilium, the Physician, Patient and Res Publica Litteraria in Early Modern Consilia Literature

Abstract

In this part of the book, the knowledge obtained from the works of selected physicians is systematized and supplemented. The initial chapters focus on the circumstances that accompanied the process of creating an individual consilium, such as selection of a counsellor, his remuneration, or the way of handing over the consilium. It is shown which circumstances affected the whole process. Next, great attention is paid to subsequent formation of collections or anthologies of consilia. The paratext material documenting the work of the editors, their financial or advertising intentions is extremely important. The necessity of a broader approach to the study of all early modern medical genres connecting the Respublica iatrica from the 16th century to the 19th century is emphasized.

Keywords: consilium, editors, collections, anthologies, paratext material, communication

3.1 Creation of Consilia

3.1.1 Selection of Counsellors – Faculty of Medicine or Renowned Physician?

When an attending physician needed the aid of expert advice, he had two options from which to choose: to contact a medical institution (faculty of medicine, collegium medicum), or a specific specialist. Situations in which an attending physician or patient himself contacted a faculty of medicine with a request for assistance were evidently not in any way uncommon. The process of preparing consilia by the medical committee of a faculty

Divišová, Bohdana, *Medical Case Studies (Consilia medica) of the Early Modern Period*.
Taylor & Francis Group, 2022
doi: 10.5117/9789463723640_ch03

is documented in the Hessen Medical Code from the year 1616, which was treated by S. Salloch in her work.[1] It states that when a dean receives a written request for a consultation or visit, he should call either all or at least several members of the committee, read the letter and write a protocol of the opinions of each colleague and his own together with an expert analysis. A designated physician was then supposed to prepare a consilium for the patient according to the joint resolution for which he was supposed to receive double the fee as compared with his other colleagues. In the event that a visit to the patient was requested, the patient's attending physician was supposed to describe the case orally or in writing beforehand. After this, according to the wishes of the patient or his relatives, the dean designated one or even several physicians, who visited the patient together and shared their findings with the council. In the cited work, the author notes that according to prescribed regulations, the patient had to contact the entire medical council, but it is not likely that he could not contact an individual physician.[2]

A tradition of ordering consilia from a team of professors of a faculty of medicine is confirmed by the numerous consilia of D. Cornarius in which his colleagues from the faculty in Vienna participated,[3] or a consilium from Solenander's anthology, which for all the professors of the faculty of medicine in Leipzig was signed by its dean, Wolfgang Meurer.[4] The existence of this practice in Italy is documented by a consilium by B. Vettori of the Paduan faculty, which was written "with the consent of all participants," and many of Montanus's consilia proposed after advising with other physicians.[5] And even the consilia of G. Capivaccia or V. Trincavelli were supplemented by the opinions of their faculty colleagues.

The second option for an attending physician was to seek out one concrete physician and a couple of questions appear in connection with this. In the selection of an institution, its success and renown clearly played a role, but were the criteria in the selection of an individual counsellor the same? Could

1 Salloch, *Das hessische Medizinalwesen*, 88.

2 Ibid., 89.

3 Cornarius, *Consiliorum medicinalium tractatus*, 83, Cons. X. "The noble lad was ... brought to a gathering of Viennese physicians ...;" 101-2, Cons. XII. "The Viennese physicians gathered, ... whose names are recorded at the end of this document;" 139, Cons. XX. "... the consultation took place in Vienna among these physicians ..."

4 Solenander, *Consiliorum medicinalium sectiones*, Sect. III., 225-8. Cons. V. "Sequitur Lipsensium sententia. In Melancholia ... consilium Clariss. Viro D. Achatio a Veltheim, a Professoribus Lipsensibus."

5 Victorius, *Medicinalia consilia*, 1556, 5r., Cons. I.; Montanus, *Consultationum medicarum opus*, 1, Cons. I.; 150, Cons. LIX., 390, Cons. CLXII., etc.

the patient involve himself in the selection, or did the attending physician have to have the patient's consent in order to request advice from a colleague? What role did price or personal relations and contacts between physicians play here? Some of these questions can be answered relatively easily. "Noble sir, requested by the patient himself, I will discuss my consilium for his treatment briefly with you."[6] Thus C. Guarinoni proved that patients could of course propose counsellors. In a similar manner, even though it does not seem that way according to the opening words, R. Solenander found a counsellor. "When I started treating Elizabeth, Nikolaus's wife, a few days ago ... I proposed that they select one of ... the medical council of your town as a collaborator ..., so that with our combined efforts and joint consilium, ... more easily defeat the disease. For which Nikolaus wanted most to consult with you, whose thoroughness and skill he has already made use of many times before ..."[7]

The patients of other physicians also certainly asserted their will, but much like today we can assume that attending physicians preferred to turn to colleagues with whom they already had some experience. The numerous consilia correspondence between C. Guarinoni and A. Samperolio, who was Guarinoni's friend and successor in the role of personal physician to the Duke of Urbino, may serve as an example. Their close relationship is, among other things, evident in the fact that in the consilia Guarinoni informed Samperolio not only of his successes, but also confided in him concerning his problems at the court in Prague.[8] In one of the consilia of J. Wittich for a change, the counsellor and attending physician were related.[9] However, obtaining a contact for a particular counsellor could take place within the framework of the scientific community. In one of his consilia, T. Mermann recommended one of his friends to well-known Augsburg physician Adolf Occo: "... Godefredus Seeg wrote a scholarly book about this spring ... for this reason ask this excellent physician; I can provide the contact because I know him personally."[10] Although Mermann did not arrange consilia for his friends, if the consilium of a particular specialist were requested, he would likely approach finding a contact in this manner. Unfortunately, we

6 Guarinonius, *Consilia medicinalia*, e.g. pg. 61, Cons. XLII.

7 Solenander, *Consiliorum medicinalium sectiones*, Sect. I., 66, Cons. XVI.

8 Guarinonius, *Consilia medicinalia*, 736, Cons. DCXIIII., "You know me and so will easily believe me ..."; 771, Cons. DCXX. "Concerning my quarrel, know ..." etc.

9 Wittichius, *Medicorum consilia*, 541-58. Cons. LXXIIII.

10 For more see Mermannus, *Consultationes*, 526. Cons. XXVIII. Flemish physician Godefrid Versteegh (Steghius, Steeg, d.1608) worked as the personal physician of Bishop of Würzburg J.E. von Mespelbrunn and subsequently Emperor Rudolf II.

cannot present a specific example, where a student contacted his professor because of consilium. Looking for advice firstly from or through a friend, relative or teacher is entirely natural even today, so it was undoubtedly the same in the early modern period.

The physician Bucher was also friends with J. Fernel, whom he asked to evaluate a consilium prepared by the renowned Jacobus Sylvius for his patient.[11] Fernel obliged, criticized the consilium of his colleague from the faculty and even sent his own consilium with comments. We cannot say to what extent this corresponded to the ethics of the time, but as we can see, it was also possible to obtain a new counsellor in this way.[12] And here we have touched upon the issue of collaboration and antagonism among physicians. Let us take a small detour and recall that consilia collaboration was not always without its difficulties. Recall the comment of G. Capivaccio, who completely tore the consilium of his colleagues to pieces with the statement that their treatment would certainly not work.[13] The co-workers with whom Capivaccio disagreed were the no less renowned university professors Bernardino Paterno, Girolamo Mercuriale and Girolamo Fabrici d'Acquapendente. The titles of some consilia testify to the disputes of C. Guarinoni with his colleagues: "Consilium created after lengthy disputation against important physicians, especially Capivaccio ...;"[14] or "Defense of the above-mentioned opinion."[15]

Other conflicts because of the treatment of patients involved not only collaboration between colleagues. Mentions, which often appear in consilia, testify to the continuous conflict between physicians with medical degrees and unorthodox groups of healers, hidden behind the labels: dabblers, Empiricists, Paracelsists, Jews, Agyrtae, medicastri, "wise old women" or even representatives of religious orders. The discrediting of these groups directly inspired the publication of Matthaeus's collection-anthology, but denunciations can also be found in the consilia of other physicians.[16] Guarinoni complained that his patient "... committed himself into the hands

11 Fernellius, *Consiliorum liber* 1582, 13v., Cons.12.

12 In the case of renowned Bohemian physician and astronomer Tadeáš Hájek z Hájku (Haggecius, Nemicus, d. 1600) a similar breach of collegiality contributed to the taking of legal action. For more see Hayck [sic], *Actio medica*, 66-7.

13 Capivaccius, *Opera omnia*, 964-5, Cons. XX.

14 Guarinonius, *Consilia medicinalia*, 409, Cons. CCCLXXXVII.

15 Ibid., 353, Cons. CCCLI.

16 Matthaeus, *Consilia medica*, 87-8. "At that time, a certain Jew used flattery to gain favor, ..."; 105. "It would take a long time ... to list here all of the nonsense and foolishness of those, who consider themselves empiricists ...".

of known arrogant people [Paracelsists] ..., "[17] and "Jewish Empiricists" or an "Anabaptist pseudo-physician" interfered in the treatments performed by Cornarius.[18] It should however be noted that these non-university-educated healers were not always viewed entirely negatively. The most inconsistent view was of Empiricists, who had "the most problematic label of all [charlatans]."[19] Even in a consilium one can discern a struggle that took place between an irresponsible, dangerous medieval Empiricist and an early modern Empiricist, who courageously uses his reason, experience, and observations. R. Solenander was not in any way afraid of trying medicines proposed by an Empiricist and moreover, did not feel aggrieved that the patient sought help from someone so "inferior": "After writing my consilium, a Jewish ... Empiricist contributed ... medicines, which – since I quite approve of them – I wanted to share with supporters. These are ..."[20] Guarinoni also appreciated empiric medicines several times in the treatment of lues, as we shall note.[21]

3.1.2 Payment for Consilia – Money or a Gift?

In connection with the creation of the consilium, it is also essential to examine the financial compensation aspects. The question of payment or the overall financial situation of physicians in different countries and periods has not yet been satisfactorily addressed. Of course, exceptions exist regarding individual cases or physicians, cities, or groups of physicians.[22] This topic even appears in the Hessian Code: participants in an advisory group were each to receive one gulden, the physician, who eventually created the written form of the consilium, the resulting resolution of the council,

17 Guarinonius, *Consilia medicinalia*, 713, Cons. DLXXXVII.

18 Cornarius, *Consiliorum medicinalium tractatus*, 39. Cons. II. "... ab Empiris Iudeis ... male curatos ...;" ibid., *Observationes*, 8 "... consilio malo ... cuiusdam Anabaptistae Pseudomedici ..."

19 Gentilcore, *Medical Charlatanism*, 61.

20 Solenander, *Consiliorum medicinalium sectiones*, Sect. I., 19, Cons. IIII. "Post hoc meum consilium datum Iudaeus ... Empiricus ... medicamenta quaedam suppeditavit, quae cum ego satis probem, volui studiosis ea communicare. Ea haec sunt. ..."

21 For more see chap. 4.4. of this work.

22 For example, the financial situation of physicians in Florence of the 14th and 15th centuries was addressed by K. Park, for more see Park, *Doctors and Medicine*, 152-7; similarly for Bologna Pomata, *Contracting a Cure*, 98-100. Information concerning the financial situation and "salary" of individuals can be obtained about J. Fernel, for more see Sherrington, *The Endeavour*, 99. From the newer works e.g., Ofenhitzer, *Praxisalltag*, 105-15. R. Weston covered this topic for later consultation literature. For more see Weston, *Medical Consulting*, 35-42. Nevertheless, even here there are more questions than answers.

was to receive double the payment.[23] Other European faculties of medicine certainly handled the financial compensation for the council of professors in a similar manner, but the fees probably varied. One can assume that the greater the renown of the faculty and professors, the more the customer had to pay. But how was it with payments for a consilium which an attending physician or patient ordered from a renowned figure? Was it usual to pay for the advice in advance? Did the fee vary depending on the length of consilia, wealth of the patient or difficulty of the case? And was the payment always monetary?[24]

Answers to some of the above-mentioned questions can be found thanks to ever-growing knowledge about the communication networks of the modern "Res publica litteraria" of which "Res publica medica" was also an integral part. The sharing and exchange of information and gifts became the main buttress of the European scientific community. A. Quaranta accurately captured the process of mutual exchanges of gifts in her study: "... a gift triggered long-term exchanges and established trusting relationships that could in turn translate, ..., into auxiliary tools for scientific studies (information, drawings, books) or in a more strictly material (pharmaceutical substances, money loans) or professional kinds of aid (interceding with a printer, giving advice on a patient's treatment)."[25] In addition to the cases mentioned in previous chapters, documentation that even consilia became items of exchange is provided by "epistolae medicinales." Although correspondence could involve individuals who were strangers to one another, they were generally friends – and who else do you ask for medical assistance, if not a friend?

The important Humanist A. Dudith turned to his friend, Opava physician W. Raphanus, with his health problems quite regularly. "My year-old son fell from the table yesterday, ... abandoned by a careless nurse, suffered a wound on the upper part of the tongue ... What do you order us to do? ... Do you think that he may speak poorly due to that wound? Advise quickly, my doctor!"[26] Immediately in the subsequent letter he asks Dudith for advice

23 Salloch, *Das hessische Medizinalwesen*, 91-2: Each participating physician was to receive one gulden for the consilium, and the patient or his family could designate the number of consulting physicians, thus limiting them to 2-3 and the ordinarius. For an in-person visit, each received half a gulden, the ordinarius a full gulden and at night the amounts were double.

24 E.g., personal physicians in continual service received part of their pay in kind. For more ibid., 49-52. This is also confirmed in the employment contract of physician O. Rovereti. For more detail see Divišová, "Krátká zpráva," 154.

25 Qaranta, "Exile Experiences," 89-90.

26 Crato, *Consiliorum liber tertius*, 262.

because of the treatment of his daughter.[27] Raphanus was however not the only physician with whom Dudith consulted: "I like your consilium, which arrived here not long ago..."[28] This is how he reacted to the aid from Lorenz Scholz with whom we are already well acquainted. It is not likely that Dudith paid these and probably even other physicians for the consilia sent to him in cash, but rather (as even today commonly between friends) he repaid them with a gift in the form of a book, uncommon medicine, or intermediation of other contacts within the scientific community. Even physician A. Samperolio could "repay" his friend C. Guarinoni for dozens of consilia in a similar manner and it appears that in addition to informing him about events at the Court of Urbino, he took care that Guarinoni (who intended to return to his native Italy) was not completely forgotten there. As F. Mauelshagen summed up "...the rules of commercium litterarium demanded reciprocity, but neither the 'currency' of a return gift nor the date of its 'payment' were laid down. Obligations were largely unspecified and rested on good faith."[29] However, this trust was not completely limitless, everyone involved knew that "... networks were the field within which moral pressure could be exerted. This does not only become obvious in situations of conflict; in fact, it was a permanent feature underlying friendly interaction, ..."[30]

It is nevertheless unimaginable that all those ordering consilia were members of the scientific community and would only pay with occasional gifts or information, especially since an absolute majority of the renowned early modern physicians wrote hundreds and possibly even thousands of consilia during their lifetimes, as besides the educated physicians was confirmed by even Girolamo Mercuriale.[31] Two hundred years later in England the standard price for a consultation by mail was one guinea, but as the author of the study W. Wild noted, the amount was not fixed, the physician considered the financial circumstances of the patient as well as bonds of friendship, so a written consultation was occasionally free of charge.[32] It is certain that it was necessary to pay for consilia ordered from a collegium of a faculty of medicine or private physicians, but I have not

27 Ibid., 265.

28 Crato, Consiliorum liber quintus, 373.

29 Mauelshagen, "Networks of Trust," 24.

30 The author also gives several examples of mutual misunderstandings due to unwanted or unsolicited gifts, when expectations of reciprocity were disappointed. Ibid., 23-4.

31 Siraisi, *Communities of Learned Experience*, 27, 108. It is of course a question to what extent it was a consilium of the faculty council and to what extent a private one.

32 Wild, *Medicine-by-Post*, 184.

found any mention of financial remuneration, let alone for example, the negotiation of the amount of the fee based upon the wealth (or lack thereof) of the patient or length of the consilium in any consilium published in print or other written correspondence between physicians of the researched period.[33] Precise information can be discovered by chance and more likely in manuscripts. For example, in the year 1603, a scribe from the Royal City of Rakovník (Rakonitz) sent to a Prague physician a request for a consilium for his sick wife and together with a urine sample, he enclosed an advance of one ducat for treatment and a tolar for medicaments.[34] Whether this amount represented the usual norm cannot be confirmed or refuted due to a lack of sources. We can just summarize that consilia were a significant component in the solidification of the network of contacts and in addition to money, other forms of "capital" were also no less important motivations for their composition.

The last link in the process before the practical use of consilium was its delivery to the patient or attending physician, which depended upon the postal connection and its speed. According to authors L. Brockliss and C. Jones, who focused on the history of medicine in France, the boom in remote consultations depended on transportation and although remote consultations were known in the 17th century, in their opinion they only began to pay off in the following century, when the postal service improved.[35] In England during the same period, patients on the contrary expressed concerns about the unreliability of the postal service and of improper behavior of postmen, who supposedly stole money intended for the payment of consultations from envelopes.[36]

Although contact via written correspondence was a cornerstone of the "Res publica litteraria" throughout the entire early modern period and was far more extensive than previously thought, one cannot say anything more precise about the methods and speed of transporting consilia.[37] Although, for example, there had been a functioning state post office in the German lands since 1595, the most common method of transmitting information was evidently the dispatching of a special messenger as documented

33 This situation was similar in later times, see Brockliss, "Consultation by Letter,"111, note 45.

34 Winter, *Šat, strava*, 312-3.

35 Brockliss and Jones, *Medical World*, 536.

36 Wild, *Medicine-by-Post*, 183.

37 R. French assumes that medieval consilia traveled faster than diseases and thanks to them, physicians could prepare perhaps for the outbreak of epidemics, which is not very likely. For more see French, *Canonical Medicine*, 278.

by numerous mentions of "tabelarii" in consilia and correspondence.[38] Moreover, university professors could occasionally use their migrating students to carry correspondence, while physicians of rulers had access to court courier services. The method and speed of the transportation of consilia in the 16th century, like the question of their financial (or other) compensation, however are not yet sufficiently researched and the same applies to latter centuries.[39] However, as noted by F. Mauelshagen in his study "...a time gap between letter and response, and consequently between gift and return gift, was an unavoidable structural element of every *commercium litterarium*."[40] Obtaining information concerning the means of postal transport, just as the speed of the exchange of correspondence, depends on notes preserved by chance and the care with which physicians dated correspondence. As an example, we can use a letter-consilium of E. Gockel, who from Schaffhausen on July 16th of 1692, informed his consultant colleague that he had just received his letter sent by the colleague on July 8th from Düsseldorf.[41] More detailed research may uncover interesting information about more than the land route connections. A work of an important Dutch physician of the 17th century even captures the route of a request for a consilium (for a pregnant syphilis patient) from the Norwegian port of Kristiansand to Amsterdam, which in the year 1697 took just under a month.[42] Although many editors of consilia collections published in print in the 17th and 18th centuries were very meticulous with regards to dates, in this area, the study of archival materials will evidently be more beneficial, as indicated by the already mentioned modern studies. More in-depth and thorough research is the foundation for learning about all aspects not only of consilia, but also the other related genres at which we will now take a closer look.

38 More about the development of postal connections (not only) in Germany see Fontius, "Post und Brief," 269. The more common practice of sending letters through a selected person is proven by the example of Solenander, *Consiliorum medicinalium sectiones*, 493, Cons. XVII. "Yesterday around breakfast your messenger arrived. I will send him at three in the afternoon at the earliest..."

39 More detailed study may uncover information not only about overland postal connections. A work by an important Dutch physician of the 17th century for example even captures the route of a request for a consilium (for a pregnant luetic patient) from the Norwegian port of Kristiansand to Amsterdam, which took under a month in the year 1697. Blancardus, *Opera medica*, 522.

40 Mauelshagen, "Networks of Trust,"23.

41 Gockelius, *Gallicinium medico-practicum*, 549. "Hoc momento literas a D. D. Brunnero Dysseldorpio accepi, datas 8. Julii." Scaphusii d. 16. Julii, 1692.

42 Blancardus, *Opera medica*, 522.

3.2 Real Consilia Versus Related Genres

Related genres have already been mentioned in connection with the establishment of consilia literature in the course of the 14th and 15th centuries. The generation of these older genres (for example plague consilia, regimina et al.) continued, but in the 16th century many of these older types underwent significant transformations brought on by new philosophical movements (for example, Neo-Hippocratism), and especially the closer connection with the practical activities of physicians. In particular, the types of humanistic professional medical literature which were based upon personal observations and recorded the personal experience of physicians, began to develop and gain ground ever more strongly.[43] However, let us keep in mind that the borders between genres were very fluid and definitions imprecise (according to today's professional criteria). At the beginning of the 17th century, the physician Antonides van der Linden categorized genres in his bibliography into consilia, consultations, observationes, historiae medicae, epistolae medicinales, and responsa, but their differentiation in actual medical practice was not at all so unequivocal.[44] This can even be easily documented among the selected representatives of consilia literature.

"Consultationes medicae" gained particular importance in the medical literature of the 17th and 18th centuries, but this designation was mostly perceived as a synonym for the term consilia. In da Monte's collections of consilia, "consultations" appear with the lengthy title: "List of medical consultations..., in which one hundred others have been added to all those consilia published earlier."[45] Moreover, as noted by G. Pomata, due to the inclusion of detailed, eye-witness descriptions of the treatment of fevers and instructions for writing "histories," da Monte's consilia significantly approach the direction of the genre of "observationes."[46] A similar convergence of terms is documented by the collection of C. Guarinoni, whose editor titled the collection "Consilia medicinalia," while the individual advices are then

43 This topic is covered generally in the anthology of works of Siraisi, *History, Medicine, and the Traditions*. For more on consultation letters see ibid., 63-105.

44 Lindenius, *De scriptis medicis*, Consilia, 532-3; Consultationes, 533; Casus medici, 534; Epistolae, 478-80; Observationes, 490, 534; Historiae medicae, 533, Responsa, 480. For more on the separation and formation of medical genres in the 16th century see Pomata, Praxis Historialis, 105-46.

45 Montanus, *Consultationum medicarum opus ... In quo ad consilia omnia prius edita, ... accesserunt ...*

46 Pomata, "Praxis Historialis," 128-9. "Da Monte's Consultationes, collected and published posthumously by his students, indicate the transition from the old genre of the consilium to the new observational approach."

called "consultation," or the collection of T. Mermann titled "Consultationes ac responsiones medicae,"about which its editor remarks in the introduction: "I collected these *consilia* from various manuscripts..."[47] "Responsa" appeared in the dedication of the fourth edition of Fernel's collections of consilia, where it is mentioned that they have published "... responses of Jean Fernel, which are usually called consilia."[48]

In early modern medical literature, observations became one of the most important and progressive forms of professional literature and according to G. Pomata, even partially supplanted consilia.[49] The description observations of an interesting case of a disease or treatment was close not only to consilia, but also to "unusual cases" (historiae rarae) and the later "curiosities" (curiosa) or "miraculous recoveries" (mirabilia).[50] Just as in the case of consultations and responses, even observations could be connected with consilia. In the anthology of R. Solenander there are many observations. Some were designated as consilia, while elsewhere the author realized the differences in the genres.[51] In these cases observations appear as "Pro Consilio" (instead of consilium).[52] The editor chose the same approach for the categorization of Solenander's medical correspondence, where a letter to a friend is in one place termed a consilium and elsewhere as "pro consilio."[53] Unlike in the case of Solenander, Diomedes Cornarius placed "Observationes medicinales" and "Historiae admirandae rarae" separately after his consilia. As already mentioned, not all his consilia are "real" and due to their form, many of them belong rather in the section of "Observationes." This is for example evidenced by the eighth consilium, which captures the

47 Guarinonius, *Consilia medicinalia*. In addition to this, this author regularly used "cura" as a synonym for consilium. For more see ibid., 324. "Cura, vel consilium;" 443 "Consilium, vel cura." Mermannus, Consultationes. "Collegi autem consilia ista ex variis manu-scriptis..."

48 For more see Fernelius, *Consiliorum medicinalium liber, ... consultationum selectus*, 1589, a2r. "... Ioannis Fernelii ... responsa, quae Consilia vocari solent."

49 For more see Pomata, "Observation Rising," 45-80; or Pomata, "Praxis Historialis," 131. "The 'curatio' and 'observatio' were clearly the new genres that tended to replace the 'consilium,' although the latter did not disappear."

50 For more about this type of consilium also see Siraisi, *Medicine and the Italian Universities*, 226-52.

51 Solenander, *Consiliorum medicinalium sectiones*, e.g. 493, Cons. XVI. "Rara quaedam et tamen observatione digna, quae in sectione corporum occurrerunt: ..."

52 Ibid., e.g., 487, Pro Consilio XV. "Singulares aliquot observationes, quae ad consilia curandi pertinent: quarum partim ipse observavit, partim ab aliis observata ... notavit ...;" 493, Pro Consilio XVII. "Condiendi funui medicatum modus," etc.

53 Ibid. 498, Cons. XVIII. "Ad Levini Pontani, Landgravii Pharmacopolae, Epistolam, responsum de alumine ...;" 500, Pro Consilio XXI. "Clariss. Viro ... D. Gerardo Mercatori amico integerrimo ..."

approach to the treatment of a tumor over the course of several months, the death of the patient and his autopsy.[54]

A consilium could however become an integral part of an "observation"and vice versa.[55] We can borrow an illustrative example of this from another physician, Pieter van Foreest (Petrus Forestus, 1521-1597), whose works were essential for the establishment of the genre of observations.[56] For example, in Forestus's "Observationes et curationes" we can read about the case of the hernia of his brother-in-law, who described his condition in a letter in German. Forestus responded in Latin with a consilium and eventually published the entire case with results as an "observatio."[57] One could object that here the response is called a "consultation" and the communication did not take place between physicians, but instead between a physician and patient. Although we know that consultatio was a synonym for consilium, we can provide a better example. In the case of the wife of a Delft burger from the year 1563-4 that was recorded in great detail, Forestus published three consilia, which he, together with another attending physician, received from Cornelius Gemma and the personal physician to Emperor Charles V., as well as his correspondence with them, the request letters.[58]

"Observationes" had a parallel in another early modern genre called "historiae" (sometimes also "casus"), where the fundamental difference compared to classic consilia was the record of the complete case, including the successful or unsuccessful result of the treatment.[59] "Historiae" could also be added to a collection of consilia, as shown in the works of G. Ballonius, or the title of Cornarius's collections "Consiliorum medicinalium tractatus" (Treatise on Medical Consilia), where "Observationes" and "Historiae

54 For more see Cornarius, *Consiliorum medicinalium tractatus*, 73, Cons. VIII. De Aneurysmate in pectore oborto. A similar approach to the description of a "sports" injury can be found in the collection of observations; for more see ibid., Observationes, 29, XIII. De casu cum equo.

55 See Calabritto, "Curing Melancholia," 630.

56 For more see Pomata, "Observation Rising," 54; or Santing, "Pieter van Foreest," 149-69.

57 Forestus, *Observationum et Curationum medicinalium libri*, 610-2, Liber XXVII., Observatio XXI. in qua agitur de Enterocele, per modum Consultationis. "Theodorus Teylingius, Sororius meus, ... in herniam intestinalem incidit ... Cum litteris, quamquam lingua Germanica scriptis, a me consultationem petered [he asked me for advice in a letter written in German], ego Consultationem lingua latina hanc ipsam scripsi ...[I wrote the following consultation in Latin.]"

58 Ibid., 731-5, Liber XXVIII. De Mulierum morbis, Observatio LXIIII. De Mola aut sanguine crassiore, quem hydrops subsequebatur, deinde mors. Ibid., 732, "... Cornelii Gemmae Lovaniensis Consilium in casu uxoris D. Pensionarii"; 734-5, "Consilium Mathisii, Medici olim Imperatoris Caroli Quinti."

59 For more on histories in medicine see Pomata and Siraisi, *Historia: Empiricism and Erudition*; or Siraisi, *History, Medicine, and the Traditions*.

admirandae rarae" were also classified.[60] As previously noted, physicians procured copies of his consilia, either for publication, or for their own private use. Thus, they could later even add the result. This is the case of many consilia of C. Guarinoni, which were evidently originally sent as a letter to a distant recipient. This is documented by the introductory remarks of the consilium: "... in the letter of the physician, I was informed of your health ... I immediately wrote you a consilium ..."[61] The consilium itself concludes: "This [patient] became weaker, was overcome by fever and died."[62] However, if the result of the treatment of the patient (often even with a brief description of his obduction) does appear, shouldn't a consilium be called an observation or history...? It is not the objective of this study to resolve this dilemma and it can only confirm the veracity of the statement of N. Siraisi made long ago: "A full history of method and content in early modern observations and records of individual medical cases would need to explore not only the influence of ancient examples and the development of new science, but also the sixteenth-century fortuna of the consilium format."[63]

The final genre related to consilia to which we have not yet devoted closer attention, is "epistolae medicinales" (medical letters). This correspondence regarding medical topics, which was conducted among physicians and laymen, is enjoying growing interest among researchers.[64] The close connection between letters and consilia is given due to their nature and fundamental purpose to connect distant people with information.[65] Due to the fact that physicians, compared to those in other fields, focused more strongly on professional issues in their correspondence, the linking of consilia and other medical correspondence was completely natural.[66] This is confirmed by the titles of the researched collections, for example the series of "Crato's" "Consilia et epistolae,"[67] or Wittich's "Consilia, observationes atque epistolae

60 Ballonius, *Consiliorum liber secundus*, where 8 histories were printed before the consilia themselves.

61 Guarinonius, *Consilia medicinalia*, 333, Cons. CCCXXX.

62 Ibid., 334.

63 Siraisi, *Medicine and the Italian Universities*, 77-8.

64 E.g., Nancy G. Siraisi, *Communities of Learned Experience*; Ian Maclean, "The Medical Republic of Letters before the Thirty Years War," *Intellectual History Review* 18, no. 1 (2008): 15-30.

65 As an example, we can mention the extensive publication on the renowned physician T. Erastus, for more see Charles D. Gunnoe Jr., *Thomas Erastus*. Here we can find a detailed list of Erastus's correspondence, 441-62, while the existence of Erastus's numerous consilia is only briefly mentioned. Ibid., 470.

66 For more see Maclean, "The Medical Republic," 21.

67 Crato, Consiliorum liber quintus, 265-75, Cons. XL. Here we also find a demonstrative example of the linkage of regimen and consilia; a separate "regimen gravidarum" was attached to a consilium for a pregnant woman.

medicae."[68] The merging of these genres is manifested not only in the titles, but also in the contents of individual consilia or letters. In one of his consilia, C. Guarinoni describes to his friend the last moments of the life of the notable Bohemian politician, William of Rosenberg, as an eyewitness. It is of course understandable that he did not mention any medical advice or prescriptions here.[69] On the other hand, there are many letters from various authors, which except for their opening address or sentence are typical consilia. This is frequently confirmed by the correspondence attached by Scholz to Crato's anthologies.[70] In the case of Solenander, there also appears "In the course of seriously impaired health ... written letter," in which Solenander even published prescriptions, so that it again resembles a consilium.[71]

A younger German physician, Eberhard Gockel in his collection "Observationum et Curationum medicinalium" linked correspondence and consilia together in an interesting way. Regardless of the title, he terms individual cases as consilia; one of these consilia can be presented as an example.[72] In July of the year 1692, Gockel wrote a consilium for Albert Fugger and he ended his proposal of treatment with information that the patient requested the opinions of other physicians, so the author contacted his colleague.[73] Within the scope of one consilium, Gockel then published five letters exchanged with the physician concerned and this correspondence is also interspersed with individual pieces of advice from the letters of other colleagues with whom these physicians consulted independently of one another. All communication ended in December 1692 with the message that the patient had died.[74]

We could continue listing the genres related to consilia. As I. Lonie noted, a consilium required a certain discussion about the case and complexes, and thus could easily turn into a general discursive essay about the problem under discussion.[75] Treatises were attached or mixed in with consilia, which is evidenced by both the titles of collections, as well as their contents.

68 Wittichius, *Medicorum consilia*.

69 Guarinonius, *Consilia medicinalia*, 716, Cons. DLXXXXI.

70 For example, Crato, *Consiliorum liber tertius*, 394-5; 395-6; 397-8; Crato, *Consiliorum liber sextus*, 5-9. Epist. III.; 31-6, Epist. X. et al.

71 Solenander, *Consiliorum medicinalium sectiones*, 496-7. Pro Consilio XVII. In animi et corporis misere afflicta valetudine: ... scripta epistola.

72 Gockelius, *Gallicinium medico-practicum*, Centuria II., 544, Cons. LXXIV.

73 Ibid., 545. "Et quia praefatus ... Patiens etiam aliorum clarissimorum Medicorum de suo affectu sententiam scire desiderabat, idcirco ... Domino Johanni Jacobo Wepfero, Medico ... morbum hunc cum omnibus circumstantiis per literas notificavi, qui mihi per sequentes respondit."

74 Ibid., 562.

75 Lonie, "The 'Paris Hippocratics'," 172.

One example is the first edition of Trincavelli's consilia, which included treatises under the name of consilia.[76] From the aforementioned facts, we can see the evident continuation in the lack of a clear definition of genres in the 16th century, whose interconnection – aptly labeled by M. Calabritto as "hybridization" – is absolutely inseparable.[77] In order to lead an apt discourse, it is essential not to specialize in one genre. As a summary of the literature, we can paraphrase the statement of N. Siraisi, which was cited above: A complete examination of early modern consilia would require not only the study of classical examples and scientific developments, but also a large number of observations, various forms of medical records, treatises, and most of all medical correspondence.[78]

3.3 Collections and Anthologies

3.3.1 Numbers of Consilia in Collections and Anthologies

The number of consilia in anthologies and collections varies greatly in scope: from the nine consilia of a particular Matthaeus anthology to collections of several dozen consilia mostly rendered in great detail even to extensive publications with several hundred individual entries. However, as already stated above, the result of the count does not have to be unequivocal: there are officially 279 in the third publication of Trincavelli's consilia, but if we include the contributions of his consulting colleagues, their number comes close to seven hundred. The numbers for real collections penned by one author are not as high, but nevertheless the numbers of consilia from Mermann and de Baillou climbed to almost three hundred. The collection of Cristoforo Guarinoni stands out among all the selected authors with over six hundred consilia. Moreover, these consilia only represent a part of the total unfortunately to us unknown and inestimable number of consilia, which he wrote or possessed. Guarinoni's publisher confirmed this with a note that he left out many consilia, and even mentioned the name of the consulting physician whose consilium was left out.[79] The same also documents the

76 Trincavellius, *Consiliorum Libri; Epistolarum Medicinalium Libri tres*, 111v., Cons. LXXXVIII. Sermo de Cordis affectibus; 112v., Cons. LXXXIX. Sermo de animi defectu.

77 Calabritto, "Curing Melancholy", 629.

78 For more on the definition and typology of different types of medical records see Hess and Schlegemilch, "Cornucopia Officinae," 11-38.

79 Guarinonius, *Consilia medicinalia*, 549. This note brings into question whether all of the consilia in the collection were really written only by Guarinoni.

unknown fate of 400 consilia of Jean Fernel and almost certainly applies to the other authors and their works.

3.3.2 How Consilia Were Collected for Publication

A collection or anthology of consilia consists of more or less numerous independent literary works. Understandably, obtaining and collecting a sufficient number of consilia necessary for the compilation of a book sometimes posed a problem. On the other hand, paper was expensive and consilia could just have been printed thanks to the thrift of the printer. R. Solenander, who was called to print his consilia in order to fill extra pages, clearly expresses this in his preamble.[80] A similar situation also appears in the 1597 republication of Fernel's consilia to which the consilia of other Parisian physicians and "observationes" of F. Valleriola were added with the explanation from the editor that he considered it better to at least print something rather than leave the pages blank.[81]

The preambles of the selected collections and anthologies have already indicated several ways to collect a sufficient number of consilia. The most common was probably the method demonstrated by L. Scholz, whose call to send the consilia of German physicians enabled him to compile a record number of anthologies.[82] These consilia evidently most often came from the hands of attending physicians, who kept them even after the recovery of the patient, or the relevant physicians obtained them through their copying and sharing among colleagues, as implied in the correspondence between Monau and Scholz.[83] Reiner Solenander, who asked his patient directly to copy his consilium and send back the original (or copy) of his manuscript, dealt with this more simply.[84] However, as the editor of Mermann's collections informs us, consilia also represented a commercial product and could be purchased.[85] Another source of consilia were students, who could record them during theoretical instruction (if their professor used them for this purpose), or capture orally presented consilia during practical instruction

80 Solenander, *Consiliorum medicinalium sectiones*, 2r.-2v.

81 Fernelius, *Consiliorum medicinalium libe*, 1597, 171.

82 Crato, *Consiliorum liber*, 4r. "Again, I beg all those devoted to medical science not to refuse to entrust to me the consilia of German physicians, if they possess them ..."

83 Ibid., 365.

84 Solenander, *Consiliorum medicinalium sectiones*, 497, Cons. XVII.

85 Mermannus, *Consultationes*, Dedicatio, without pagination. "I collected these consilia from various manuscripts here and there, either randomly purchased or borrowed from friends or sent to me kindly from elsewhere."

in the course of actual hospital rounds, which was the case with da Monte's consilia from the Hospital of St. Francis.

The estates of deceased physicians also included consilia, most often the consilia of colleagues, which the concerned physician either ordered, copied, exchanged, or purchased. However, in Guarinoni's posthumously published collection, many of his own consilia appeared, sometimes including information concerning the fate of the patient. Thus, a physician could make copies of his consilia, or – like Solenander – ask the recipient to make a copy. However, if we look at even the number of consilia known to us, it is evident that the production of such a number of sometimes quite long literary works (among many physicians this certainly involved at least one thousand items) and possibly in several copies, required a lot of time. Mermann's complaint about day-long copying, as Thiermair recalls, bears witness to this, while a similar lament from the renowned professor of the Paduan faculty, Girolamo Mercuriale, was also recorded.[86] Evidently, not every patient or attending physician was willing to make a copy, let alone send the original back. Where did these physicians find the time to make copies, while performing their professional duties (treating patients)?

One of the possible explanations was captured in a letter from a professor of the faculty of medicine in Padua, da Monte, when he wrote to his friend and student Crato: "After reading your letter ... I quickly ... dictated [a response] because of the account of those, who wrote it; [they were] very educated young men, your countrymen."[87] Although this sentence refers to the dictation of a letter, there can be no doubt of a similar approach to consilia, especially since "epistolae medicinales" is one of the most closely connected genres. There is nothing new under the sun in that university professors made use of the assistance and services of students. It is evident that for the sake of speed, perhaps due to the need of "accounts" in the form of several copies due to record-keeping, or the intended inclusion in collections and publication, letters and evidently even consilia were dictated – in this case to willing German students. They were then certainly not prevented from recording the opinions of their teacher for private use in their educational materials, which they eventually brought home. Remember that students from German countries contributed significantly to the preservation and provision of the consilia of all three Paduan professors whose collections were included in the study. Many of them were already professors at universities north of the Alps at the time of the publication of the consilia.

86 Ibid., 6v.; to Mercuriale see Siraisi, *Communities of Learned Experience*, 27.

87 Montanus, *Consultationum medicarum opus*, 6r.

However, how did physicians who held important positions, for example at court, and were sought-after counsellors, but did not have the option to use students, approach this? We can even find an answer to this question either in the correspondence or consilia. One of the best documentations is again an account of the editor F. Thiermair, who confirmed that Mermann dictated his consilia and letters to his assistants.[88] The mentioned "amanuenses" may have been paid scribes but were much more likely young physicians in training. In Italy at this time, it was already a long-standing practice that new graduates practised under an experienced colleague for a period of time. For example, according to a decree of the Paduan Faculty of Medicine, a graduate was allowed to open his own practice only after one year as an intern.[89] In accordance with the Italian example, this practice also became the norm in Europe north of the Alps, as documented by many specific cases.[90] Mermann's editor also mentions that his father, physician Thomas Thiermair, was "at the service" of Mermann in his final years.[91] A mention concerning the physician Seehauser, who "at some time practised under the same Mermann" hints that multiple interns were to be found around Mermann.[92] It is likely that they provided Mermann some reciprocal services, which may also have included work on copies of consilia.

In a similar way, we may interpret a mention in the dedication of commentaries to Aristotle from Cristoforo Guarinoni, who sent one of the young men, "who I usually have with me due to educational interests," to Padua.[93] The existence of such interns would also explain the position of the often-mentioned Augustinus Lucidus in Guarinoni's consilia. Guarinoni expressed his favor to this physician, supported him and used his influence to get Lucidus admitted to the Imperial Court in Prague.[94] Guarinoni allowed him to

88 Mermannus, *Consultationes*, 6v.

89 For more see Cipolla, *Public Health*, 4.

90 For example, Georg Handsch accompanied Andreas Gallus and Pietro Andrea Mattioli. For more see Michael Stolberg, "Empiricism in Sixteenth-Century Medical Practice," 490. The Tyrolean physician Hippolytus Guarinoni was trained by his father, the former imperial physician Bartholomeo Guarinoni. For more see Guarinonius, *Grewel der Verwüstung*, 712.

91 Mermannus, *Consultationes*, 6v. "… Thomae Thiermairio p.m. qui ultimis annis Mermanno utpote amanuensis adstitit …"

92 Ibid., Cons. XIV., 197. "… ita ex M.S. D. Seehauseri, qui olim apud eundem Mermannum praxin exercebat." [… according to a manuscript of … Seehauser, who at one time trained in practice under Mermann.]

93 Guarinonius, *Sententiarum Aristotelis*, 4.

94 Guarinonius, *Consilia medicinalia*, 736, Cons. DCXIIII. "Ad haec designavit Doctorem meum Augustinum Lucidum ipsi Aulae in Physicum et ei dictum voluit se id fecisse, quo mei diutius curam haberet." [To this [C.M] designated my doctor Augustinus Lucidus as the court physician and wanted him to be told that he did so in order to maintain my services for a longer time …]

participate in the treatment of one of the most import nobles of the Kingdom of Bohemia, William of Rosenberg, and in the course of this, Lucidus requested a consilium from Guarinoni, evidently from the position of a subordinate.[95]

These facts raise much speculation. Did all renowned physicians have such assistants around them? How many physicians could a renowned practitioner train at once? Did a physician-newcomer need recommendations, nepotism, or an amount of money in order to serve as an intern under a colleague of high standing? Finding the answers to these (and other) questions will evidently depend on archival study. The contents of a pleading letter in which the 43-year-old and highly regarded physician Georg Handsch, dissatisfied by the earnings of his practice in Prague, offered his services to renowned colleague Pietro A. Mattioli, may indicate something.[96] For room and board and 100 Rhenish guilder per year he promised to continue the translation of Mattioli's Herbarium into German and would also handle all of the written administrative duties.[97] In connection with the creation of consilia the question arises as to whether requests for consilia were among the written administrative duties. Yet another intrusive question presents itself: if so, many renowned physicians complained about a lack of time and the incessant writing of responses, what prevented a busy counsellor from delegating the preparation of written responses to a younger colleague? For a junior physician it would represent invaluable experience and the senior celebrity could only check, correct and sign the proposed treatment in the consilium. If a consilium was prepared for an employer by an experienced physician such as G. Handsch, was he allowed to sign it as well? We cannot yet answer these questions but can only state that high-status physicians were commonly surrounded by several assistants or younger colleagues, who for the opportunity to gain experience or for a salary assisted them and thanks to whom many consilia were evidently preserved for us.

3.3.3 Editors, their Work and Dedications

All of the collections and anthologies of consilia which I have included into my probe, were regardless of the life dates of the authors, published

95 Ibid., 703, Cons. DLXXXIII.; 697, Cons. DLXXVII. Ad Augustinum Lucidum Doctorem ... De Prorege Boemiae Guglielmo Rosimbergio ... [To the excellent physician Augustinus Lucidus. Concerning the Bohemian Viceroy William of Rosenberg]. In addition to Rosenberg, Lucidus also treated another of Guarinoni's patients, the Spanish Ambassador in Prague, Gullielmo de San Clemente, for whom he wrote a consilium. For more see *Consilia diversorum Medicorum*, fol. 149-158.

96 Winter, *Doktoři a lékaři*, 6.

97 Letter is dated April 26, 1561.

(with but two exceptions) in the second half of the 16th century and at the beginning of the 17th century. The questions of printing and editors, especially of collections and anthologies published posthumously, have already been mentioned. Grateful students are first among the editors, who contributed to the preparations of publications. The consilia of da Monte, Capivaccio, Fernel and essentially even Mermann were edited by their students (at least the discussed publication). In the other cases, relatives took action – Trincavelli's first publication was arranged by his son Bernard, while a similar situation can be seen in the case of Wittich, and the consilia of de Baillou were published by his nephew. Only Crato's consilia were published by his devoted friend Scholz, while the person behind the publication of the largest consilia collections of Guarinoni is unknown.

It is very difficult to uncover editorial changes in collections, which were not prepared for publication by the author himself. Fortunately, this happened in many preambles, but nevertheless one cannot tell whether or not it was an observed rule. In the previous chapters, it was mentioned that many editors of consilia were very conscientious and continuously informed readers of their changes in the text. This applies to the publisher of da Monte's consilia of Crato, who "with great effort and care corrected, added what was missing and removed the distorted," and Mermann's editor Thiermair, who informed readers of all of his major modifications right in the title of the book.[98] He informed about his changes even in detail in for example the following manner: "Attention: medicines were not given in this consilium ... I replaced them with what Mermann usually prescribed in similar cases."[99] Thiermair also made translation changes, and – like Crato – with a sigh testified that editorial work was always demanding of time and patience.[100] On the other hand, the editor and also translator of Fernel's consilia, G. Capellus swore in the dedication that he had changed nothing in the consilia.[101]

In the re-editions and publications where the intention of the editor was to improve the usefulness of the collections and to systematize their contents, changes of an entirely different kind and especially greater in scope appear. This was demonstrated by an analysis of two editions of Trincavelli's

98 Montanus, *Consultationum medicarum opus*, A3v.; or 126 "Hoc in loco poteram aliquid monere de Correctione ..."; Mermannus, *Consultationes*, ... "partim ex Germanico et Italico idiomate in Latinum versae. Partim in multis locis, annotationibus et remediis succedaneis, auctae: ... in libros octo distinctae."

99 Ibid., 41r. Cons. III.

100 Ibid., 5v.

101 Fernellius, *Consiliorum liber* 1582, a II v.

consilia, where the printer as well as editor Waldkircher implemented a very radical reorganization along the lines of "practica" works and made changes to consilia, from which "... that, which in addition to persons and certain circumstances had no greater benefit for medicine, was removed."[102] However, even translations of consilia from a national language into Latin could represent major editorial changes. These are confirmed in da Monte's, "Crato's," Mermann's, Wittich's and Fernel's collections, and it is difficult to determine whether the translation led to any material shift. Moreover, some consilia could be translated by a layman, who was not necessarily completely proficient in the medical terminology of the time or formulations.[103]

Dedications of individual books are an important part of paratext materials and for this reason, they received closer attention.[104] An absolute majority of the examined works was for understandable reasons dedicated to the patrons and employers of either the authors themselves, or of their editors or printers. This was the case of da Monte's consilia dedicated by Crato to the senators of Wroclaw, and the collections of Trincavelli, Venusti, Solenander, Mermann, Wittich, and de Baillou, whose editors tried to ingratiate themselves with their employers. Lorenz Scholz surprisingly dedicated all his volumes to his friends and acquaintances from the correspondent community – professors of the faculties of medicine from German-speaking regions, which was evidently an expression of his proclaimed effort to make the German nation more visible. One can find different dedications in Victorinus's collections, the publication of which was supposed to immortalize the healing arts of the renowned Mattioli (even though we have already mentioned that this evidently was not the only reason), and the third publication of Trincavelli's collections, which through its dedication was probably supposed to influence the so honored person as an intercession or even a "bribe."

No less interesting is the supposed motivation that moved the author or editor to publish the consilia. The most common reason was a natural effort to contribute to the recovery of patients and provide a helping hand to an unknown colleague with advice from a renowned expert, as mentioned by for example Vettori, Solenander and editors Capivaccio or de Baillou. The assistance of students of medicine represented a major motivation, as emphasized for example in the preambles to the consilia of da Monte,

102 Trincavellius, *Consilia Medica* 1587, 4r.-4v.

103 E.g. Wittichius, *Medicorum consilia*, 1. "... began to translate German consilia into Latin, which was completed after his death by Master Erasmus Hedanus."

104 For more on the significance of paratext materials see Maclean, *Logic, Signs*, 42-3.

Crato, Cornarius, Solenander and Fernel. Authors and publishers however must have been aware how important a segment of the market with books precisely students represent, and the recommendation of a book as a suitable learning aid often contributed to it being quickly sold out.[105] Accentuated in the same manner was the desire to help society, as expressed by Crato, Trincavelli's publisher or Venusti. Other motives include an effort to contribute to generations of humanity, not deprive humanity of valuable knowledge and an overall need to help anyone else, as expressed by Scholz and the editors of Fernel, da Monte, Guarinoni or Wittich; of course, esteem for a teacher appears several times as one of the reasons for publication, which for example Crato highlighted in the publication of da Monte's consilia, furthermore, friendship expressed by Scholz and Fernel's editor, or filial love expressed by Bernardo Trincavelli. Particular motives for publication were expressed by Matthaeus, defending his professional honor, Solenander's motivated publisher, who had extra pages, and the physician Thévart, who gave the reason for the publication of de Baillou‘s consilia as the genre being little known in France.[106] However, the Frankfurt publisher of Capivaccio's consilia, I.H. Beyer, who in a disparaging manner mentioned the quality of the previous Italian and French editions, had a special reason.[107]

In the preambles, regardless of whether their author was the editor, printer or the physician himself, the main reason for the publication of collections was assistance: assistance to individuals (the patient and his bumbling attending physician), assistance to groups – beginning, still inexperienced physicians or medical students during their studies, and not least help to the entire wider society and all of humanity.[108] A however less apparent and proclaimed reason was an effort to demonstrate membership in his scientific community and contribute to the growth of awareness concerning a common sense of belonging. Assisting the "Respublica iatrica" was also mentioned at the beginning of the 17th century by the publisher of de Baillou's

105 For more see Maclean, *Learning and the Marketplace*, 63, 70.

106 Under similarly random conditions, the council of another famous physician, F. Valleriola, was also printed, where we will read after the dedication of the councils of physician S. Petreus. "...I have gathered these consilia, the remnants of my father, with great reverence and I entrust them to your learning ..." The printer's note follows: "Because we have a few blank pages left, we have supplemented them with the advice of a learned doctor F. Valleriola." Fernelius, *Consiliorum liber*, 1597, 153-61.

107 Capivaccius, *Opera omnia*, 4r.

108 These reasons also appear in latter consultation literature of the 17th-18th centuries and in publications of collections of medical letters. For more see Weston, *Medical Consulting*, 23, 26, 41 et al.; Maclean, "The Medical Republic," 22.

consilia, F.I. Thiermair.[109] However, in the preface to the publication of his own consilia a half century later, this same physician somewhat cast doubt upon all of these reasons.[110]

3.3.4 Anthologies, Advertising and Book Printers

Anthologies, meaning groupings of consilia written by multiple authors, clearly predominate among the editions of medical consilia studied, and even volumes titled collections by their editors and published under the name of one of the physicians may in fact be anthologies. This is not only the case of the third publication of "Trincavelli's" consilia, but also of others: da Monte, Capivaccio, Cornarius, Solenander, Wittich or Matthaeus and in part also Fernel. This could have happened for several reasons: firstly, the use of the name of the physician, who recorded the decision-consilium of the entire faculty (or even other) collegium of physicians in writing, or the name could have served as advertising. This could apply to da Monte's collection, where the listed co-consultants were professors of note, but had lesser renown than da Monte. The anthologies published by Scholz, which mention that they are the consilia "of Crato and other excellent physicians," arouse similar suspicion, but while the name of Crato jumps out from the page due to the size of the font and in some publications even because of the red color, the note concerning the inclusion of the consilia of other physicians is hardly noticeable. One might assume an attempt by the publisher to make use of a famous name for advertising and thus increase sales.[111] This assumption is also confirmed by two supplementary Hanoverian publications in which the names of Crato and Scholz were used, even though they were already deceased for many years.

The competition in the literary market was strong, but collections of consilia were evidently popular and sought-after items, which is even confirmed for example by Reiner Solenander, who in his preamble states that the sale of all copies of the first edition is the reason for the republication.[112] The popularity and financial profitability of the genre is also supported by the fact that publications of the collections of at least six of the fifteen physicians (Vettori,

109 Ballonius, *Consiliorum liber tertius,* a II r.-v. About the process of forming belonging to the scientific community, for example Findlen, "The Formation of a Scientific Community," 380. An example is given in the natural sciences. Ibid., da Costa Kaufmann, „Empiricism and Community," 408-11.

110 See chap. 2.11. of this work.

111 For more concerning the approach, practices and competition among publishers see Maclean, *Scholarship, Commerce,* 101-3.

112 Solenander, *Consiliorum medicinalium sectiones.*

Trincavelli, Guarinoni, Cornarius, Mermann and Wittich) were paid for by a printer or bookseller. The publications of Vettori's, Trincavelli's and Guarinoni's were taken care of by one of the most renowned publishers of medical literature of the period: Valgrisi, Waldkircher and Meietus, and it would be no surprise if this were also determined for the cases where the person financing the publication is not mentioned. The consilia thus fully confirm the finding of I. Maclean that "the market was sustained largely by speculative publication financed more by publishers or patrons than by authors themselves."[113]

The majority of consilia anthologies and collections were published in print only after the deaths of their authors, so conjecture concerning the physicians' interest in their publication exclusively because of advertising, as presented until now in some historical works, does not correspond to reality.[114] Only six physicians (Vettori, Venusti, Scholz, Solenander, Cornarius, Matthaeus) were able in any way participate in the editorial work, promote the taking into consideration of their opinions on the arrangement, or influence the inclusion or modifications to individual consilia and the overall appearance of the collections. All of this however with respect to the requirements of the publisher, the not yet well researched customary practices and relationships between the author, editor and printer, and of course the distance between the printing location and the location of the author. To what extent could Lorenz Scholz, who practiced in Wroclaw, influence the actions of the printer of his and "Crato's" collections published in distant Frankfurt, or how did Diomedes Cornarius from Vienna influence the printing of his book in Leipzig? The most logical explanation of the mutual communication between the printer and editor or author is (other than presence in person) written correspondence.

The importance of medical letters for mutual professional communication between individual representatives of the "Res publica medica" is well known but is however not mapped in detail. It is here that, besides personal and professional discussion, future research may also uncover documentation concerning contracts and agreements regarding the publication of books. A chance reference in unpublished correspondence between J. Crato of Krafftheim and his colleague in imperial service, Bartholomeo Guarinoni indicates that medical correspondence can reveal all kinds of things about

113 Maclean, *Learning and the Market Place*, 78, or idem, *Scholarship, Commerce*, 101-3. These claims correspond more or less to the findings regarding publications of physicians' letters, even if these appear to be less attractive financially. For more see idem, *The Medical Republic*, 22.

114 This is confirmed by numerous consultations, where treatment failure and patient death are recorded.

publishing activities. In one of the letters, B. Guarinoni mentions difficulties with the publication of a book of another imperial physician, Giulio Alessandrini.[115] "I saw how much you did for Julio's book. ... Julio's son and I spoke with Joannes Aubrius and if we are able to judge, his father-in-law Andreas Wechel will probably not be interested in this..."[116] A similar mention also appears in one of Crato's letters to the Nuremburg humanist, J. Camerarius. This time, Peter or Jacob Monau was taking care of the publication of Crato's but, however, not to Crato's complete satisfaction. "Nuremburg and Frankfurt publishers are now fighting over my book. This was achieved by Mr. Monau, who assumes too much authority over it."[117] These references illustrate the importance of the research of all related early modern genres because the above-mentioned letter belongs to a collection of "epistolae medicinales" and documents the interconnection of the scientific community of the period and the mutual sharing of scientific works.[118]

3.4 Patients

Many historians, starting with the authors J. Agrimi and Ch. Crisciani, have noted that in consilia literature the patient did not quite stand at the center of attention. Even though there was generally no room for them in the highly scholarly correspondence of experts, we will attempt to summarize the information that consilia can provide us with concerning patients. First

115 For more on B. Guarinoni and his correspondence with J. Crato see Divišová, "Ärzte mit den Nachnamen Guarinoni," 89-101.

116 "Pro Julii libro quantum E.V. effecerit, vidimus. ... Magnus et Ecc. Julii filius, et Ego, cum Joanne Aubrio locuti sumus, et quantum animadvertere potuimus, difficile Andreas Vechelius eius socer, huic rei dabit operam ..." Biblioteka Uniwersytecka we Wroclawiu, Sign. R 248/51.

117 Crato, *Consiliorum liber quintus*, 379. "Litigant nunc de eo Typographi Norinbergenses et Francofurtenses. Haec concivit D. Monauius, qui nimis magnam potestatem sibi in meum libellum sumpsit."

118 This fact is also confirmed in the study by I. Maclean, who with regards to the availability of books before the creation of market catalogs states: "...correspondence with colleagues and references in printed books were the principal ways of learning about recent production; when a doctor found out about a book, he then sought to borrow it from a local source, or get some patron to buy it for him." For more see Maclean, *Learning and the Market Place*, 75. However, as the presented references from correspondence show, a no lesser source for procuring new books was a friend participating in the affairs of "res publica litteraria." This fact is confirmed most convincingly by the request of the noted humanist, A. Dudith, directed at physician L. Scholz: "If you have any manuscript or print, ...please send it... If you obtain any nice treatise related to philosophy or medicine, please do not hesitate to share it with me." Crato, *Consiliorum liber quintus*, 376.

of all, the titles used clearly show that the patients of all of the mentioned physicians came from the upper or even the highest classes of the population and this fact is also confirmed by a survey of other consular collections.[119] Of course, exceptions can be found even among the most renowned counsellors, for example, members of his household or the court of an important figure.[120] One must consider whether renowned counsellors could have had more "poor" patients, but that editors preferred to publish consilia for wealthy patients. It is also possible that correspondence between a counsellor and personal physician paid by a rich client was more likely to be printed than a consilium sent directly to a less affluent patient. Nevertheless, it is more logical that only members of the upper classes could afford to pay for the services of celebrity physicians, so we can generalize that the more renowned and higher status the physician, the more renowned and higher status his patients. The renown of a counsellor is documented by the greater number of those across Europe interested in his consilia. Unsurprisingly, these included professors at the University of Padua, da Monte and Capivaccio, or the renowned J. Fernel, who epitomized the combination of two of the greatest possible careers – personal physician to a ruler and a concurrent university career. Guarinoni's patients were also from throughout Europe, which was due not only to the composition of the Imperial Court, where representatives of all the countries of the monarchy worked as courtiers, but also by the presence of diplomatic representatives of many European powers. Municipal physicians cared for on average the rather well-situated members of the middle classes. These differ significantly from patients in hospitals, whose treatments were recorded through observation by students and who could not afford the care of a physician. This fact is most evident in Monte's consilia intended for a group that in the past stood outside the center of any attention: children from impoverished circumstances.

Among the recipients of the counselling, male patients clearly predominated. M. Calabritto also noted a significant predominance of male patients in the consultations she examined, but it cannot be confirmed that this could be due to "reasons of privacy and decorum."[121] As will be shown below, early modern physicians did not suffer from shyness, and let us recall that the inclusion of the consilium in the press often depended on chance. The

119 M. Calabritto devoted herself to the consultations of prominent professors G. Mercuriale a G.C. Claudini. See Calabritto, *Medicina practica, consilia* and the illnesses," 74.

120 E.g. Guarinoni, *Consilia medicinalia*, 532, Cons. CCCCLXIV. "Pro ...Illustrissimi Cardin. Caraffae Domestico..."

121 Calabritto, "*Medicina practica, consilia* and the illnesses," 74.

conclusion that women were in the minority among the recipients is obvious (and probably corresponds to reality), however, this impression cannot be generalized, as it is based on only a few printed collections and most of the consultations lie unexplored in manuscript form in the archives.

The names of patients appear very irregularly, sporadically in general, among the individual authors and consilia. In many cases the patient was not specified because "consilia were not about patients" and the editor considered the name unimportant. Patients themselves could consider their treatment by a renowned physician as presenting their own importance and wealth and thus may not have protested against the publication of their names.[122] Nevertheless, as documented by some preserved and researched "work performance contracts" between patient and physician, many employers in the 16th century made medical confidentiality a condition.[123] This of course was especially true with regards to rulers, whose state of health was an important component of the intrigues and calculations of top-level politics.[124] However, if the consilia were printed after the death of the physician (or even the patients), this obligation of confidentiality may not have been valid any longer. In conclusion, a note on the dates and locations at which consilia were composed: both appear as sporadically as the names of patients. However, it seems that consilia recorded by students during hospital visits, or consilia sent to patients in the form of a letter (that is, "real consilia") bear the dates and locations of their writing more often than others.

3.5 A Physician's Career and his Consilia

Seven of the selected physicians tied their professional careers, or at least the main part of their lives, to the teaching of students at one of the faculties of medicine: Of the six selected Italian physicians, only two – Venusti and

122 For more on this kind of advertising see Pomata, "Praxis Historialis," 125. By contrast, the successful post-battle-of-the-White-Mountain Czech politician and confiscator Pavel Michna of Vacinov was furious with his attending physician M. Borbonius of Borbenheim due to the consilium concerning his case, because it involved the treatment of Michna's impotence. For more see Gellner, *Životopis lékaře Borbonia*,173-4.

123 For more see Salloch, *Das hessische Medizinalwesen*, 41, 138. Even in much later times, confidentiality was not completely automatic and although a gentlemen's codex was assumed, physicians published cases of their patients without taking their feelings into account. For more see Wild, *Medicine-by-Post*, 125, 129.

124 Salloch, *Das hessische Medizinalwesen*, 41-2. The significance of the knowledge of the state of health of the monarch can be documented by the records of ambassadors at the court of Rudolf II. For more see Bůžek and Marek, *Smrt Rudolfa II.*, 5-25.

Guarinoni – were not professionally connected to the academic world, while the other four, Vettori, da Monte, Trincavelli and Capivaccio, were important professors of medicine at the universities of Bologna and Padua. With the exception of Capivaccio, all had experience running a municipal practice, to which only Venusti remained true. For Guarinoni the position of personal physician was typical, while the main calling of the others became teaching: B. Vettori, G.B. da Monte, V. Trincavelli, J. Fernel, D. Cornarius, G. Capivaccio, G. de Baillou.[125] Some of them however can also be counted among an even larger group of physician-counsellors, who looked after the health of an important ruler or noble. In addition to C. Guarinoni, J. Crato, R. Solenander, J. Wittich, T. Mermann and J. Matthaeus, this group could also include J. Fernel, G. de Baillou, and D. Cornarius. This finding is not in any way surprising since rulers logically tried to enlist the best physicians into their service and those, as is customary even today, are found (or should be found) among the instructors at the faculties of medicine of universities.[126]

Only two of our selected sample belonged to the final and lowest-status group in comparison with both of the previous two, the municipal physicians: A. M. Venusti was a municipal physician in Trieste his entire life and L. Scholz practiced in Freistadt and Wroclaw. Nevertheless, if we take a closer look at the concise biographies of the others, we find that an absolute majority of those included in our study held the position of a municipal physician or private general practitioner. The renowned da Monte practised in Brescia, V. Trincavelli in his native Venice, C. Guarinoni in Verona, J. Crato first in Verona and eventually in his native Wroclaw, R. Solenander in Lucca, D. Cornarius in Trnava, J. Wittich practised in Sangerhausen and Eisleben and finally became a municipal physician in Arnstadt and J. Matthaeus practised in Hannover. However, based on the information available, it is not possible to judge whether all of these physicians practiced independently, or were just undergoing training by accompanying an experienced colleague as was the custom. It should be noted that based on the (limited) dates on consilia, it is evident that these physicians began to be asked for consilia to a greater extent only after they had climbed several steps higher up their career ladder. This can be documented by the number of consilia of Reiner Solenander, an ordinary physician at the sulfurous spa in Lucca and the consilia of Reiner

125 Thomas Mermann was active at the university in Pisa, but according to references only taught philosophy.

126 The relationships between personal physicians and university professors and the linkage of both positions were treated in the greatest detail in Salloch, *Das hessische Medizinalwesen*, 101-4.

Solenander, the personal physician of the Dukes of Jülich. This impression may be misleading due to a range of circumstances (for example, the low and selective number of consilia published in print, the small number of researched authors). Nevertheless, concerning professional medical works, I. Maclean stated that "both town physicians and court doctors produced learned work, the majority of new publications came from the pens of university teachers", and a more detailed study of consilia literature may in the future show that this genre is the proverbial exception that proves the rule.[127] The likelihood of this also increases with the analogous opinion expressed by G. Pomata concerning a closely related form of literature called "observations."[128]

3.6 Paralipomena and Summary

The previous chapter concludes the first part of the book dedicated to consilia literature as a whole. The detailed presentation of the works of representatives of 16th-century medicine has allowed us to examine the content, form and manner of publication of consilia in the 16th and in part also the following two centuries. I have attempted to arrange and compile the results into clear sections devoted to the circumstances and process flow in which consilia originated. Not all aspects received the attention they deserve, and many have not yet been mentioned. These include, for example, the increasing tendency for editors to prefer compiling anthologies. This trend can be observed starting at the end of the 16th century and is understandable since obtaining consilia by a range of authors is easier than collecting a large number of consilia by a single author. There did not have to be any link between the randomly collected consilia and their authors. This is even documented by the words of Augsburg physician G. H. Welsch that accompanied the publication of 400 consilia from 15 physicians of the 16th and 17th centuries: "I arranged the consilia of various physicians that I found with me and had never yet been published."[129]

The common link could have become work at the same university, professing a certain manner of treatment (Galenists or Paracelsists), or belonging to a nationality or speaking a language. The linking element could also have

127 Maclean, *Learning and the Market Place*, 63.

128 For more see Pomata, "*Observation Rising*," 59.

129 Welschius, *Curationum Exotericarum Chiliades*. Praefatio ad Lectorem, sine pag. „... medicorum variorum collectas in ordinem redegi, quae omnia apud me Mssta. et nunquam edita exstant." Welsch's consilia were released posthumously by his friend L. Schröckius, who was – like Welsch – a member of the Academia Leopoldina. See Welschius, *Curationum propriarum*.

become a patient whose treatment generated multiple consilia from several physicians, which is the case of the previously mentioned Matthaeus's anthology for the Duke of Baden, Ernst Fridrich, or the consilia collection for the Spanish Ambassador in Prague, Guillémo de San Clemente.[130] Whether the religious confession of authors played a role in the selection of consilia for a collection, cannot be said with certainty.

In the anthologies of physicians of the 16th century to which this study is first and foremost dedicated, differences in approaches exist. In Italian anthologies published under the name of a renowned physician, either the separate opinions-consilia of all physicians who collaborated as co-consultants, are presented, or all of the members of a faculty council are signed under a joint consilium. Anthologies that originated in German lands are mostly anthologies in the contemporary sense of the word, i.e. sets of different consilia of various authors, one of whom – usually the most famous – bestowed (knowingly or not) his name upon the anthology.[131] Essentially only four books of the selected sample are collections of the consilia of a single author, while all the other eighteen books are anthologies containing dozens of consilia and the names of many physicians whose works were not originally part of the study.[132]

Anthologies compiled in German-speaking lands are characterized by several particular attributes: in addition to stronger expressions of patriotism, which I. Maclean noticed even in "epistolae medicinales," it is notable that their editors did not hesitate to include in their publications not only the consilia of renowned personal physicians and university professors, but even those of lesser-known physicians. Furthermore, in "German" anthologies, we find the consilia of representatives of Italian and French medicine (thanks to which ten consilia of the French physician G. Rondelet, which were not published elsewhere, were published), but consilia of German physicians were not published in Italian or French anthologies.[133]

The final observation is the gradual increase in the numbers of republications. This does not mean just entire anthologies, but also individual consilia. The original consilium, taken out of the original collection, repeatedly appeared in new anthologies compiled at various times by various editors and publishers.

130 Manuscript sign. D. D. II. 22 in the Strahov Library contains the copies of the consilia of eleven physicians, predominantly renowned professors of the Paduan faculty of medicine.

131 The proverbial exception among them is the work of D. Cornarius.

132 It is however necessary to note that Guarinoni's authorship of all the consilia in the collection is not completely without any doubt.

133 I. Maclean explains this fact by the strongly expressed medical superiority of Italian correspondents. For more, Maclean, "The Medical Republic," 23-4.

Due to the facts mentioned above, it is clear that in the event of interest in obtaining exact data concerning the number of preserved consilia of one specific physician, difficult heuristic work awaits researchers. They will have to determine not only information about the reeditions of one specific collection or anthology, but also determine the number of other professional works in which individual consilia appear, removed from the original collection. Remember however that editors could adjust the structure and shorten certain parts of the consilium or even leave out the name of the author in different editions.

However, despite the growing compilation trend, no editor was evidently enticed to cover the topic of the treatment of a single specific disease with an anthology of consilia. Only publishers of the sixth "Crato's" anthology lined up 32 consilia on the treatment of catarrh from various authors.[134] A separate anthology devoted to one disease has not been discovered yet, even though it would be surprising if such a publication were not attractive for medical students and junior physicians. Nobody took advantage of the opportunity to collect into one volume as many consilia as available on the treatment of ocular diseases, melancholy, infertility or the French disease, even though "morbus gallicus" was a disease with which every early modern physician had to contend. In the 16th century this disease afflicted every social class of the population, including the highest and had a chronic course with repeated attacks and manifestations on various parts of the body and organs. Since lues also appeared in the above-mentioned collections of the authors selected, I will attempt to make use of consilia on the treatment of this disease in order to both acquaint the reader more closely with the disease itself and take a look at actual consilia. Against this background, some interesting facts, particularities of consilia literature, as well as points of similarity, which all early modern case history literature has in common, will emerge more clearly.

Bibliography

Ballonius, Gulielmus. *Consiliorum medicinalium liber secundus*. Paris: Iacob Quesnel, 1636.

Ballonius, Gulielmus. *Consiliorum medicinalium liber tertius et postremus, item paradigmata et historiae morborum ob raritatem observatione dignissimae*. Paris: Iacob Quesnel, 1649.

Baschin, Marion, Elisabeth Dietrich-Daum, and Iris Ritzmann. "Doctors and Their Patients in the Seventeenth to Nineteenth Centuries." In *Medical Practice, 1600-1900*.

134 Crato, *Consiliorum liber sextus*, 1-126.

Physicians and Their Patients, edited by Martin Dinges, Kay Peter Jankrift, Sabine Schlegemilch, and Michael Stolberg, 39-70. *Leiden: Brill-Rodopi, 2016.*

Biblioteka Uniwersytecka, Wroclaw, Odd. rekopisow, corresp. of J. Crato of Krafftheim, sign. R 248/51.

Blancardus, Stephanus. *Opera medica, theoretica, practica et chirurgica.* Utrecht: Guilielmus et Jacobus van Poolsum, 1714.

Brockliss, Laurence, and Colin Jones. *The Medical World of Early Modern France.* Oxford: Clarendon Press, 1997.

Brockliss, Laurence. "Consultation by Letter in Early Eighteenth-Century Paris: The Medical Practice of Etienne-Francois Geoffroy." In *French Medical Culture in the Nineteenth Century,* edited by Ann la Berge, and Mordechai Feingold, 79-117. Amsterdam: Rodopi, 1994.

Bůžek, Václav, and Pavel Marek. *Smrt Rudolfa II.* [The Death of Rudolf II]. Prague: Nakladatelství Lidové noviny, 2015.

Calabritto, Monica. "Curing Melancholia in Sixteenth-Century Medical Consilia between Theory and Practice," *Medicina nei Secoli (Journal of the History of Medicine)* 24, no. 3 (2012): 627-64.

Calabritto, Monica. "*Medicina practica, consilia* and the illnesses of the head in Girolamo Mercuriale and Giulio Cesare Claudini. Similarities and Differences of the Sexes," *Medicina e Storia* 13, no. 4 (2006): 63-83.

Capivaccius, Hieronymus. *Opera omnia ... qua editione, tum Capivaccii plurima typis hactenus novum vulgata in lucem proferuntur.* Frankfurt am Main: Paltheniana, 1603.

Cipolla, Carlo. *Public Health and the Medical Profession in the Renaissance.* Cambridge: Cambridge University Press, 1976.

Consilia diversorum Medicorum circa nervorum debilitatem Ill. D.D. Guilhelmi a PG. Clemente etc., Strahovská knihovna Kláštera premonstrátů premonstrátů [Strahov Library of the Strahov Premonstratensians Monastery], Prague, sign. D. D. II. 22, fol. 149-158.

Cornarius, Diomedes. *Consiliorum medicinalium habitorum in consultationibus ... Tractatus.* Leipzig: Michaël Lantzenberger, 1599.

Costa Kaufmann da, Thomas. "Empiricism and Community in Early Modern Sciences and Art: Some Comments on Baths, Plants, and Courts." In *Natural Particulars. Nature and the Disciplines in Renaissance Europe,* edited by Antony Grafton, and Nancy G. Siraisi, 401-18. Cambridge (MA): The MIT Press, 1999.

Crato a Kraftheim, Ioannes. *Consiliorum et epistolarum medicinalium liber primus.* Frankfurt am Main: Andreae Wecheli heredes, 1591.

Crato a Kraftheim, Ioannes. *Consiliorum et epistolarum medicinalium liber quintus.* Frankfurt am Main: Andreae Wecheli heredes, 1594.

Crato a Kraftheim, Ioannes. *Consiliorum et epistolarum medicinalium liber secundus.* Frankfurt am Main: Andreae Wecheli heredes, 1592.

Crato a Kraftheim, Ioannes. *Consiliorum et epistolarum medicinalium liber sextus.* Hanau: haeredes Ioannis Aubrii, 1611.

Crato a Kraftheim, Ioannes. *Consiliorum et epistolarum medicinalium liber tertius.* Frankfurt am Main: Andreae Wecheli heredes, 1592.

Dinges, Martin, and Vincent Barras, eds. *Krankheit in Briefen im deutschen und französischen Sprachraum 17.-21. Jahrhundert.* Stuttgart: Franz Steiner Verlag, 2007.

Divišová, Bohdana. "Ärzte mit den Nachnamen Guarinoni – Alle die Kaiserlichen Guarinoni", *Studia Rudolphina* 11 (2011): 89-101.

Divišová, Bohdana. "Krátká zpráva Ottaviana Roveretiho (1556-1626), lékaře Rudolfa II". [A Brief Report of Ottaviano Rovereti (1556-1626), Physician to Rudolf II.]. *Dějiny věd a techniky* [*History of Sciences and Technology*] 48, no. 3 (2015): 151-73.

Fernelius, Ioannes. *Consiliorum medicinalium liber quadringentarum consultationum selectus.* Turin: Gio. Dominicus Tarinus, 1589.

Fernelius, Ioannes. *Consiliorum medicinalium liber, cui accesserunt Responsa quaedam.* Leiden: Thomas Soubron et Moysen de Prez, 1597.

Fernellius, Ioannes. *Consiliorum medicinalium liber. Ex eius adversariis quadringentarum consultationum selectus.* Paris: Aegidius Beysius, 1582.

Findlen, Paula. "The Formation of a Scientific Community: Natural History in Sixteenth-Century Italy." In *Natural Particulars. Nature and the Disciplines in Renaissance Europe,* edited by Antony Grafton, and Nancy G. Siraisi, 369-400. Cambridge (MA): MIT Press, 1999.

Fontius, Martin. "Post und Brief." In *Materialität der Kommunikation,* edited by Ulrich Gumbrecht, Ludwig Pfeiffer, and Monika Elsner, 267-79. Frankfurt: Suhrkamp, 1988.

Forestus, Petrus. *Observationum et curationum medicinalium sive medicinae theoricae et practicae libri XXVIII.* Frankfurt am Mein: Paltheiana, 1602.

French, Roger. *Canonical Medicine. Gentile da Foligno and Scholasticism.* Leiden: Brill, 2001.

Gellner, Gustav. *Životopis lékaře Borbonia a výklad jeho deníků* [*The Biography of Physican Borbonius and Explanation of his Diaries*]. Prague: Česká akademie věd a umění, 1938.

Gemelli, Benedino. "Die Sprache der Krankheit in der Korrespondenz von Antonio Vallisneri." In *Krankheit in Briefen im deutschen und französischen Sprachraum 17.-21. Jahrhundert,* edited by Martin Dinges, and Vincent Barras, 67-77. Stuttgart: Franz Steiner Verlag, 2007.

Gentilcore, David. *Medical Charlatanism in Early Modern Italy.* Oxford: Oxford University Press, 2006.

Gockelius, Eberhardus. *Gallicinium medico-practicum, sive Consiliorum, observationum et curationum ... centuriae duae cum dimidia,* Ulm: Georgius Wilhelmus Kühnen, 1700.

Guarinonius, Hippolytus. *Grewel der Verwüstung der menschlichen Geschlechts.* Ingolstadt: Andreas Ungermair, 1610.

Guarinonius, Christophorus. *Consilia medicinalia.* Venice: Thoma Baglioni, 1610.

Gunoe Jr., Charles D., *Thomas Erastus and the Palatinate. A Renaissance Physician in the Second Reformation*, Leiden: Brill 2011.

Hayck [sic], Thaddaeus ab. *Actio medica adversus Philippum Fanchelium* [sic] *Belgam.* Amberg: Michael Forster, 1596.

Hess, Volker, and Sabine Schlegemilch. "Cornucopia Officinae Medicae: Medical Practice Records and Their Origin." In *Medical Practice, 1600-1900. Physicians and Their Patients, edited by* Martin Dinges, Kay Peter Jankrift, Sabine Schlegemilch, and Michael Stolberg, 11-38. Leiden: Brill-Rodopi, 2016.

Kay Peter Jankrift, Sabine Schlegemilch, and Michael Stolberg, eds. *Medical Practice, 1600-1900. Physicians and Their Patients.* Trans. Margot Saar. Leiden: Brill, 2016.

Kinzelbach, Annemarie, Susanne Grosser, Kay Peter Jankrift, and Marion Ruisinger. "Observationes et Curationes Nurimbergenses. The Medical Practice of Johann Christoph Götz (1688-1733)." In *Medical Practice, 1600-1900. Physicians and Their Patients, edited by* Martin Dinges, Kay Peter Jankrift, Sabine Schlegemilch, and Michael Stolberg, 169-87. Leiden: Brill-Rodopi, 2016.

Lindenius, Ioannes Antonides. *De scriptis medicis libri duo.* Amsterdam: Iohannes Blaev, 1637.

Lonie, Iain M. "The 'Paris Hippocratics': Teaching and Research in Paris in the Second Half of the Sixteenth Century." In *The Renaissance of the Sixteenth Century,* edited by Andrew Wear, Roger French, and Iain Lonie, 155-74. Cambridge: Cambridge University Press, 1985.

Maclean, Ian. "The Medical Republic of Letters before the Thirty Years War," *Intellectual History Review* 18, no. 1 (2008): 15-30.

Maclean, Ian. *Learning and the Market Place. Essays in the History of the Early Modern Book.* Leiden: Brill, 2009.

Maclean, Ian. *Logic, Signs and Nature in the Renaissance. The Case of Learned Medicine.* Cambridge: Cambridge University Press, 2002.

Maclean, Ian. *Scholarship, Commerce, Religion: the Learned Book in the Age of Confessions, 1560-1630.* Cambridge (MA): Harvard University Press, 2012.

Matthaeus, Ioannes. *Consilia medica diversorum auctorum, pro ... Ernesto Friderico, Marchione Badense.* Franfkurt am Mein: Collegium Musarum Palthenianum, 1608.

Mauelshagen, Franz. "Networks of Trust. Scholarly Correspondence and Scientific Exchange in Early Modern Europe," *The Medieval History Journal* 6 (2003): 1-32.

Mermannus, Thomas. *Consultationes ac responsiones medicae.* Ingolstadt: Joannes Phillippus Zinck, 1675.

Montanus, Ioannes Baptista. *Consultationum medicarum opus absolutissimum.* Basel: Petri, 1565.

Ofenhitzer, Franziska. *Praxisalltag in der Frühen Neuzeit. Das Rezeptdiarium von Petrus Kirstenius (1612-1616)*. Duisburg: WiKu-Verlag, 2017.

Park, Katharine. *Doctors and Medicine in Early Renaissance Florence.* Princeton: Princeton University Press, 1985.

Pilloud, Séverine. "Interpretationsspielräume und narrative Autorität im autobiographischen Krankheitsbericht." In *Krankheit in Briefen im deutschen und französischen Sprachraum 17.-21.* Jahrhundert, edited by Martin Dinges, and Vincent Barras, 45-65. Stuttgart: Franz Steiner Verlag, 2007.

Pomata Gianna, and Nancy G. Siraisi, eds. *Historia: Empiricism and Erudition in Early Modern Europe.* Cambridge (MA): MIT Press, 2005.

Pomata, Gianna. "Observation Rising: Birth of an Epistemic Genre, 1500-1650." In *Histories of Scientific Observation*, edited by Lorraine Daston, and Elisabeth Lunbeck, 45-80. Chicago: The University Chicago Press 2011.

Pomata, Gianna. "Praxis Historialis: The Uses of Historia in Early Modern Medicine." In *Historia: Empiricism and Erudition in Early Modern Europe*, edited by Gianna Pomata, and Nancy G. Siraisi, 105-46. Cambridge (MA)-London: MIT Press, 2005.

Pomata, Gianna. *Contracting a Cure. Patients, Healers, and the Law in Early Modern Bologna.* Baltimore: John Hopkins University Press, 1998.

Quaranta, Alessandra, "Exile Experiences 'Religionis causa' and the Transmission of Medical Knowledge between Italy and German-Speaking Territories in the Second Half of the Sexteenth Century." In *Fruits of Migration. Heterodox Italina Migrants and Central European Culture 1550-1620*, edited by Cornel Zwierlein, and Vincenzo Lavenia, 72-101. Leiden: Brill, 2018.

Ruisinger, Marion M. "Chirurgie im Brief. Das Beispiel de Konsiliarkorrespondenz Lorenz Heisters (1683-1758)." In *Krankheit in Briefen im deutschen und französischen Sprachraum 17.-21. Jahrhundert*, edited by Martin Dinges, and Vincent Barras, 131-42. Stuttgart: Franz Steiner Verlag, 2007.

Salloch, Sabine. *Das hessische Medizinalwesen unter den Landgrafen Wilhelm IV. und Moritz dem Gelehrten. Rolle und Wirken der fürstlichen Leibärzte.* Ph.D. diss., Marburg, 2006. http://archiv.ub.uni-marburg.de/diss/z2006/0697/pdf/dss.pdf (*12.4.2014*)

Santing, Catrien. "Pieter van Foreest and the Acquisition and Travelling of Medical Knowledge in the Sixteenth Century." In *Centres of Medical Excellence? Medical Travel and Education in Europe, 1500-1789*, edited by Ole Peter Grell, Andrew Cunningham, and Jon Arrizabalaga, 149-69. Farnham: Ashgate Press, 2010.

Scholzius, Laurentius. *Consiliorum medicinalium, conscriptorum a praestantissimis atque exercitatissimis nostrorum temporum medicis liber singularis.* Frankfurt am Mein: Andreae Wecheli Haeredes, 1598.

Sherrington, Charles. *The Endeavour of Jean Fernel.* Cambridge: Cambridge University Press, 1946.

Siraisi, Nancy G. *Communities of Learned Experience. Epistolary Medicine in the Renaissance.* Baltimore: John Hopkins University Press, 2013.

Siraisi, Nancy G. "'Remarkable' Disease, 'Remarkable' Cures, and Personal Experience in Renaissance Medical Texts." In *Medicine and the Italian Universities, 1250-1600*, edited by Nancy G. Siraisi, 226-52. Leiden: Brill, 2001.

Siraisi, Nancy G. *Communities of Learned Experience. Epistolary Medicine in the Renaissance.* Baltimore: John Hopkins University Press, 2013.

Siraisi, Nancy G. *History, Medicine, and the Traditions of Renaissance Learning.* Ann Arbor: University of Michigan Press, 2008.

Solenander, Reinerus. *Consiliorum medicinalium sectiones quinque.* Frankfurt am Mein: Andreae Wecheli heredes, 1596.

Steinke, Hubert, and Martin Stuber. "Medical Correspondence in Early Modern Europe. An Introduction," *Gesnerus: Swiss Journal of the History of Medicine and Sciences* 61 (2004): 139-60.

Stolberg, Michael. "Empiricism in Sixteenth-Century Medical Practice: The Notebooks of Georg Handsch," *Early Science and Medicine* 18 (2013): 487-516.

Stolberg, Michael. "Kommunikative Praktiken. Ärztliche Wissensvermittlung am Krankenbett im 16. Jahrhundert." In *Praktiken der frühen Neuzeit. Akteure-Handlungen-Artefakte*, edited by Arndt Brendecke, 111-20. Cologne: Böhlau Verlag 2015.

Trincavellius, Victor. *Consilia medica post editionem Venetam et Lugdunensem ...* Basel: Conradus Valdkirchius, 1587.

Trincavellius, Victor. *Consiliorum medicinalium libri tres; Epistolarum medicinalium libri tres.* Venice: Camillus Borgominerius, 1586.

Victorius, Benedictus. *Consilia medicinalia, ad varia morborum genera.* Venice: V. Valgrisius, 1551.

Welschius, Georgius Hieronimus. *Curationum exotericarum chiliades II. et Consiliorum ... centuriae quatuor.* Ulm: Schott, 1676.

Welschius, Georgius Hieronimus. *Curationum propriarum, et Consiliorum medicorum decades X.* Augsburg: L. Kronegerus et Haeredes Th. Goebelii, 1698.

Weston, Robert. *Medical Consulting by Letter in France, 1665-1789.* Farnham: Ashgate Press, 2013.

Wild, Wayne. *Medicine-by-Post: the Changing Voice of Illness in Eighteenth-Century Britisch Consultation Letters and Literature.* Amsterdam: Rodopi, 2006.

Winter, Zikmund. *Šat, strava a lékař v 15. a 16. věku* [*Clothes, Food, and a Doctor in the 15th and 16th Ages*]. Prague: J. Otto, 1913.

Wittichius, Iohannes. *Nobilissimorum ... Germaniae medicorum consilia, observationes atque epistolae medicae.* Leipzig: Henning Grossius, 1604.

4 Consilia on the French Disease

Abstract

The consilia for patients suffering from the French disease written by selected physicians are the main topic of the second part of the book. The disease is first presented in the historical context and its ontology is briefly mentioned. Attention is paid to the number of consilia for luetics in each individual collection of the selected physicians, the detail of the indications of patients, the prescription of the two most important medicines, guaiacum and mercury, and certain other specific interesting points, which could supplement known facts. Only a couple of the especially interesting consilia are analyzed in greater detail.

Keywords: humoralism, French disease, medical discourse, 16th century consilia, diagnosis, treatment

4.1 An Excursion into Early Modern Physiology and Pathology

In order to understand the early modern approach and questions regarding the pathology (not only) of the French disease, but it is also essential to familiarize oneself at least generally with humoral physiology, or according to early modern physicians, how a healthy organism functioned. An explanation of these principles can be found in every popular scientific publication devoted to the history of medicine of this period.[1] There is no need to overemphasize how important a role was played by the classic physicians Hippocrates (d.377 B.C.) and brilliant compiler and author Galen (d.199), the main originator of the theory that governed European medicine for almost two thousand years. Its foundation was the *septem res naturales*

1 To name only a selection of the many publications: Porter, *The Gratest Benefit*, 55-62, 73-7; Nutton, "Humoralism, " 281-91; Lindemann, *Medicine and Society*, 86-90; Černý, *Mor 1480-1730*, 109-291; Kusukawa, "The Medical Knowledge," 5-11; et al. For an inspirational source on a broad approach to the history of medicine of the given period see Rütten, "Early Modern Medicine," 60-81.

Divišová, Bohdana, *Medical Case Studies (Consilia medica) of the Early Modern Period.*
Taylor & Francis Group, 2022
doi: 10.5117/9789463723640_ch04

(seven natural things), which included the four basic elements (air, fire, earth, water, and according to some even the so-called fifth essence) and their corresponding qualities (hot, cold, wet, dry). This was completed with innate heat (calidum innatum) and especially the four bodily fluids (humores), which gave the entire theory its name: blood (sanguis), bile (chole), black bile (melanchole) and phlegm (flegma) of which all appendages and organs were comprised. Fluids originated in the body from food in the course of so-called concoction (concoctio), which took place in the stomach, liver and heart. The proportions of the combination of these fluids in the body (temperies) were never completely perfect and within the scope of normality, one of the fluids could predominate and thus determine the physical constitution of a person (temperamentum). This furthermore included several types of pneuma (spiritus naturales, vitales, animales), which were distributed throughout the body with the blood and variously reshape one another and their corresponding bodily and spiritual "facultates" or "vires."

The balance of the fluids in the body depended significantly upon the "sex res non naturales," meaning six non-innate things, which included activities or processes related to the surrounding environment that people need to maintain life and health: breathing (air), intake of food and fluids, excretion, sleep and awakening, bodily exercise and mental processes. Immoderate behavior would become the cause of the multiplication of one of the four bodily fluids, which then caused an imbalance in the mixture (intemperies, intemperatura, dyscrasia) and this then caused the origination of disease. However, a fluid could for a certain reason cause other pathological processes in the body, e.g. decay (putredo, putrefactio), congestion (retentio), obstruction (obstructio) and others. A concoction disorder (cacochymia) also had a negative impact on the function of the entire organism. However, external causes, most often unfavorable cosmic influences, foul air (miasma), usually due to poor hygienic conditions, but even many other factors, could also contribute to the outbreak of a disease. The renewal of humoral balance required first the evacuation of the excessive fluids, usually by means of diuretic and diarrheic preparations, perspiration, causing bleeding (most often venesection), and other surgical procedures. Very important was the subsequent adjustment to regimen (diet), which influenced the six non-innate things. Medication treatment was relatively the least important. The causes of the disease identified by the physician were treated allopathically with the respective acting preparations (mostly of plant origin).

It should be emphasized that the outline presented above is but a skeleton without the flesh, moreover a skeleton whose parts could have been variously asymmetrical. The humoral system was in its details very complex and also variable. Moreover, the 16th century was a period influenced by new movements and newly discovered (or newly translated) classical medical literature, which brought new impulses to the philosophic-medical world of thought. As a consequence of this, the Hippocratic-Galenic system was variously modified, added to and sometimes even attacked. The most well-known agitator was Philippus Bombastus von Hohenheim, called Paracelsus (1493-1541), who opposed Galenism most dramatically.[2] He and his followers are credited with expanding the use of chemical medicaments in medicine, against which dogmatic Galenists (the majority) fiercely agitated. Professor of theoretical medicine at the universities of Pisa and Turin, Giovanni Argenterio (1513-1572) was one of the other critics of Galen's physiology. He was a supporter of Paracelsian Neoplatonism, which defied not only Stoic-Galenic philosophy, but even Aristotelian Rationalism, and his controversial opinions and works caused a wave of disputes within the scientific community.[3]

Another innovator, who cannot be left out especially in connection with the French disease, is a figure we already know well, Jean Fernel. According to this French physician, a body only understood on the basis of the four fluids, especially for virulent diseases, could not be attacked. He concluded the existence of a hidden factor of a kind of occult quality, which is outside human knowledge and causes the occult root of a disease. For these diseases however instead of rational Galenic, Empiric treatment and medicines endowed with occult qualities apply. Influenced by Renaissance Platonism, he completed his system by creating his own cosmology, which explained the existence of occult matter.[4] Fernel's work and term, which he coined – fysiologia, was famous and discussed throughout Europe, but although this was original, "he did not diverge from the prevalent tradition."[5]

In connection with the French disease, one cannot omit the contribution of renowned Paduan professor of medicine Girolamo Fracastoro (1478-1553). His poem gave the name to the disease, which will be the topic of the following chapters.[6] As a supporter of atomism, he rejected the idea of hidden

2 Philippus Aureolus Theophrastus Bombastus von Hohenheim-Paracelsus (1493-1541), German physician, peripatetic mystic, founder of a new medical movement based on the study of chemical elements, study of entities and signatures, author of many new discoveries and controversial ideas. For more see e.g. Webster, *Paracelsus*.

3 For more on the innovativeness and conflicts of this figure see Siriaisi, "Giovanni Argenterio," 328-55.

4 For more see Forrester and Henry, *Jean Fernel*; or Černý, *Mor 1480-1730*, 204-7.

5 Sherrington, *The Endeavour*, 70.

6 Fracastoro, *Syphilis sive morbus gallicus*.

causes and in his works, he systematized and expanded the originally classical concepts concerning seeds of disease and several types of disease carriers: "contagium" or "infection" could spread from person to person, another carrier was the so-called "fomes," a kind of dust, which could stick to things, and the last transfer could occur at a distance.[7] As noted by M. Pelling, "... he [Fracastoro] included as contagious a range of occult influences characteristic of his period ..."[8] The principle of seeds and the spread of infectious diseases is very complicated, even more so because many physicians adapted and enriched it with their own ideas.[9]

In conclusion just a summary: The understanding of early modern physiology and pathology is made all the more complicated by the fact that every early modern physician tended to select from the competing theories and retained those that suited him according to his private interests and preferences. De facto everyone could adapt and create theories purely of their own. Although the 16th century tends to be generally considered as a kind of divide in the modern development of Western medicine and it appears to have been full of revolutionary ideas, the majority of innovations were not controversial in any way and occurred within the traditional boundaries of humoral theory. The external expression of this was the increase in professional disputes and discussions, which however took place within the framework of the scientific community.

4.2 History of the French Disease

The absolute majority of studies dealing with the history of the French disease begins in the year 1494, when an epidemic of an as yet unknown disease spread throughout Europe after the military campaign of French King Charles VIII. into Italy.[10] The question of the possible origin of this

7 For more see Nutton, "The Reception of Fracastoro's Theory," 196-243. This topic is treated in greater detail and in the context of the period in Černý, *Mor 1480-1730*, 252-4. "Fomes" was already mentioned by for example Gentile da Foligno. For more see Arrizabalaga, "Medical Responses," 51.

8 Pelling, "Contagion/Germ Theory/Specificity," 319.

9 For more detail ibid. 309-19.

10 In summary e.g. Porter, *The Greatest Benefit*, 166-7, 175; de Renzi, "The Great Pox," 146-50; Brandt, "Sexually Transmitted Diseases," 562-6; or Cunningham and Grell, The Four Horsemen, 247-80. Every year, the French disease is the topic of many expert and popular essays or monographs of European and overseas historiography, thus the studies and authors mentioned represent only a selection of these. One of the older studies is the monograph of French historian Quetel, *The History of Syphilis*. Although some opinions and facts have already been superseded,

disease attracted the attention of physicians and other researchers starting as early as the end of the 15th century. One of the greatest, today legendary disputes took place at the end of the 19th and beginning of the 20th centuries between important figures of German medicine. The defender of the so-called Columbian theory, meaning the American origin of the disease, was Iwan Bloch (1872-1922), Berlin professor of dermatovenerology and one of the founders of sexology. On the side of the pre-Columbian theory stood Leipzig professor of the history of medicine Karl Sudhoff (1853-1938) and Viennese physician Karl Proksch (1840-1923). These physicians, equipped with what today would be an extraordinary knowledge of classical languages, based their contrary assertions on detailed analysis of all mentions in classical, Renaissance and even later medical texts. To this day, this dispute has not yet been unequivocally and definitively resolved. Nevertheless, more and more scientists are leaning toward the so-called unitary theory.[11]

Opinions of the time concerning the cause of the origination of the disease and the manner in which it spreads were discussed in medical works from the very beginning of the epidemic, so many theories coexisted in the 16th century.[12] Besides being brought back from the New World, its origin was often designated as being sexual intercourse between persons afflicted with leprosy or another dermal disease.[13] Another theory searched for the specific cause in cannibalism, or in the unfavorable conjunction of planets and stars, which (similarly to the plague) disturbed the quality of the air.[14] All of these concepts were linked to the general sense that this terrible disease was sent down as punishment for crossing moral boundaries and

this monograph provides a clear overview capturing the history of the pox from its origin to the 1960s. A fundamental work on the history of the French disease of the 16th century is Arrizabalaga et al., *The Great Pox*. Especially invaluable is the opening study devoted to the historiography of the French disease with the proposed division by text, bio-bibliographic and historic traditions. Despite obstacles, like the lack of partial studies concerning the given problem, they succeeded in creating a foundational work for the study of the French disease, similar to what Les consilia medicaux by J. Agrimi and Ch. Crisciani represents for the study of consilia literature.

11 For more on the perspective on Columbian, pre-Columbian and unitary theory see e.g. Ortner, *Identification of Pathological Conditions*, 297-9; or Lindemann, *Medicine and Society*, 66-70.

12 For more concerning these opinions see Arrizabalaga, "Medical Responses," 36-42, or French and Arrizabalaga, "Coping with the French Disease," 249-51.

13 Primarily women were accused in connection with this. For more see Schleiner, "Infection and Cure through Women," 502-6.

14 For more regarding the theory concerning canabalism see Eamon, "Cannibalism and Contagion," 10-11; astrology Bloch, *Der Ursprung*, 23-32; Hayton, "Joseph Grünpeck's Astrological Explanation," 81-108; Stein, *Negotiating*, 31-4; Arrizabalaga et al., *The Great Pox*, 119-21; Cunningham and Grell, The Four Horsemen, 253-4; et al.

taboos.[15] The link of the disease to sex was evident to physicians soon after the start of the epidemic and they soon began to warn of the possible spread from mother to child, or from nurse to child and vice versa.[16] Supporters could also be found for the spread of the pox through the air, the bad smell of patients, or via dishes, worn clothing or laundry. However, all agreed according to the custom of the period that the disease prevails especially easily in those persons with an internal imbalance, which was usually caused by some fault in the so-called "sex res non naturales."

Because of its untypical symptoms, the new disease was treated from the start with mercury, which already in the Middle Ages was a commonly used preparation for dermal diseases. The side effects of the application of mercury (loss of teeth, disintegration of gums, tremors, etc.), which were considered manifestations of the disease, made the diagnosis even more difficult. Due to this, the renowned Italian physician and author of a treatise on the treatment of the pox, A. M. Brassavoli (d.1555) differentiated 234 forms of the disease based on outward symptoms.[17] At the start of the 16th century, the second most important medicine for the French disease appears – guaiac wood, the sawdust of which was used to prepare a decoction for internal use while its foam was used for an ointment for boils and sores.[18] The Fugger banking family has always been connected with the monopoly on the import of the South American guaiac to Europe, but nevertheless, newer works refer to studies that plausibly cast doubt on this assertion.[19] Guaiacum supposedly first appeared in Europe in the year 1508, and its use spread greatly in the 1520s. Both treatment preparations were in line with the humoral theory approach of the period. Firstly, they caused (for different reasons) increased perspiration, which was an integral part of the therapy, the objective of which was to remove excessive, harmful bodily fluids from the body. Other supporting treatments included hyperthermia

15 For more e.g. Stolberg, *Homo Patiens*, 49-59, chap. "Sinnsuche: Religion, Hexerei und Astrologie;" Stein, *Negotiating*, 23-9; Arrizabalga et al., *The Great Pox*, 50-4.

16 Arrizabalaga, "Medical Responses," 44.

17 Quetel, *The History of Syphilis*, 57.

18 For more concerning the history of guaiac wood and how it was used see French and Arrizabalaga, "Coping with the French Disease," 257-9; Cunningham and Grell, *The Four Horsemen*, 258.

19 This myth is disproven in the very useful work of C. Stein, for more see Stein, *Negotiating*, 101-4. Here, besides the analysis of ten early German treatises concerning the new disease, the author created an overview based on sources concerning the operation, conditions for admittance and treatment of the pox at a specialized municipal and private hospital of the Fugger banking family. The first German edition of this book, Stein, *Die Behandlung der Franzosenkrankheit*, is richer in details from the lives of patients and the broader context.

using hot baths, or time spent inside special heated barrels, purging the body through venesection, cupping, and a very strict diet.

The new disease caused terror among all classes of society and in part also among physicians.[20] The disease, whose origin was not entirely clear and long lacked a scientific name, caused a problem with respect to its classification in the Hippocratic-Galenic nosological system valid at the time.[21] The wave in which it spread from different countries and continents to others gave it more colloquial names than any other disease.[22] The situation of physicians was all the more complicated by the fact that after the initial stage of the epidemic, when the disease supposedly killed its very victims quickly (from this we have the often-used name "lues gallica," meaning the French plague), it changed into a form which caused the patient many years of suffering.[23] The virulence of the disease supposedly began to decline in the 1520s, nevertheless one of the first complete records of the course and treatment from Spanish physician Gaspare Torella from the year 1496 concludes with the "curing" of the patient (ipse perfecte est curatus).[24] Since instead of a cure one can rather assume transition into a latent stage, the transition to a chronic form of the great pox was perhaps faster than we believe. A question however remains concerning the correctness of the physician's diagnosis and the identity of the disease.

While the plague left "only" the dead in its wake, hundreds of repulsively disfigured people remained after the "French plague," and society was forced to react in some way to their existence. It became necessary to develop medical and social strategies to face this disaster and the impact on the life of the community. The first and most common approach was of course the isolation of the sick, or their expulsion from cities and towns. The expulsion

20 However, in her work, C. Stein proves that the panic of physicians was by far not as great as is usually stated in publications. For more see Stein, *Negotiating*, 22.

21 For more concerning academic medical disputes over the identification of diseases see Arrizabalaga et al., *The Great Pox*, 56-87; Arrizabalaga, "Medical Responses, " 36-45; French and Arrizabalaga, "Coping with the French Disease," 261-73.

22 For example: French, Neapolitan, Polish, Portuguese, Russian and many others. For more on the names see Porter, *The Gratest Benefit*, 193; Quetel, *The History of Syphilis*, 13; Bloch, *Der Ursprung*, 58-97, or Brown, *The Pox*, 9-10.

23 For more on the different development stages of syphilis and related diseases see Ortner, *Identification of Pathological Conditions*, 273-8.

24 For more see Arrizabalaga, "Medical Responses," 41. It involves the case of Cesare Borgia (supposedly). The descriptions of this and another four cases were designated as *consilium*. However, in the text Torella mentions that it occurred to him to recount some examples of treatment ("aliquas perticulares [sic] curas enarrare"), and thus these are not real consilia. Torella, *Tractatus cum consiliis*, fol. c4v.-d1r. (12v.-14v.).

of prostitutes, closure of brothels and baths were usually connected to this reaction.[25] The truth of this assertion is however beginning to be re-examined in modern works and it seems that the spread of the Reformation had a greater impact on the closing of brothels than the effort to combat the French disease.[26] The abolishment of houses of ill repute appeared without any connection to an epidemic of lues even in Catholic Venice and the closing of public baths in German lands was supposedly rather influenced by the high cost of wood.[27] It is however true that in many cities syphilis patients were prohibited from entering these facilities.[28]

Subsequently, specialized hospitals for syphilis patients, or at least special wards in already existing hospitals, began to be established.[29] The establishment of these facilities was at the beginning of the epidemic initiated by private parties and religious orders, while municipal authorities reacted (as usual) with a delay. In lands where the Reformation prevailed, these specialized institutions were controlled and financed rather by local authorities (e.g. city councils), while in Catholic lands the activities of orders predominated. Although the care and treatment of the disease at many of these institutions were at a good level for the time, many limitations existed for admittance into such a facility and there was naturally not room for the absolute majority of the destitute sick. However, this situation did not apply to the upper classes, as members of wealthy groups of society could afford their own physicians and in the event of problems with the treatment, the attending physician could request a renowned counsellor for advice.

By the end of the 15th century, the French disease appeared as the primary subject of many disputations and works from the pens of both physicians and laymen.[30] In every modern work on its history are presented the names of the earliest and best-known: Sebastian Brandt, Josef Grünpeck and Ulrich von Hütten among the representatives of the lay community;[31]

25 E.g. Quetel. *The History of Syphilis,* 66-7.

26 For more see Grafton et al., *New World, Ancient Texts,* 190.

27 For more see Stein, *Negotiating,* 22; McGough, *Gender, Sexuality,* 57-60. Based on the treatment of archival materials of social cultural discourse, L. J. McGough described the already endemic disease in Venice of the 16th century. Although this study is quite significantly gender oriented, it belongs among the works that should not be overlooked in the study of the history of the pox.

28 For more see Jütte. *Krankheit und Gesundheit,* 42-3.

29 For more about the development of initial reactions to the epidemic in Italy and the establishment of "Incurabili" hospitals see Arrizabalaga et al., *The Great Pox,* 171-230; Henderson, *The Renaissance Hospital,* 97-100; d'Andrea, *Civic Christianity,* 138. Concerning the situation in France see Quetel, *The History of Syphilis,* 64-6; in Germany see Jütte, "*Syphilis and confinement,*" 148-82.

30 For more see Arrizabalaga et al., *The Great Pox,* chap. "The Textual Tradition, " 4-8.

31 Quetel, *The History of Syphilis,* 13,16-9, 27-9 et al.

and Gaspar Torella, Pedro Pintor, Nicolo Leoniceno, Corradino Gilino and many others from among the physicians.[32] Even in the subsequent centuries, generations of physicians had discussions about the manner in which it spread, transmission, the type of disease and the options for its treatment, so that according to an assertion from the authors of the monograph "The Great Pox," in the 16th century lues became the second most frequent topic of medical treatises, while the plague held on to first place.[33] It has not yet been possible to verify this assertion, but nevertheless even a cursory glance at the bibliographies of the period testifies to the great interest and increase in the production of professional medical works on the topic of the French disease.[34] In Pascal Lecoq's "Bibliotheca medica" under the subtitle "Scriptores de Lue Venerea," we can count 41 names of physicians, who "... wrote separate expert treatises concerning this topic."[35] The second bibliographer, Johannes Georg Schenck, already recorded 63 names of authors of separate treatises concerning the disease and for many of them did not forget to note that their treatise was incorporated into a larger anthology devoted to this.[36] The last bibliographer, Antoninus van der Linden recorded in a section called "Specialis curatio morborum" 80 names of authors who wrote independent treatises on "Morbus Gallicus."[37]

Let us now take a closer look at the ontology of the French disease, which needs to be taken into consideration in historic research. First of all, it must be emphasized that early modern sources and descriptions cannot for historical, medical-historical and philological reasons identify with the modern picture of venereal syphilis.[38] The idea that a modern disease has its own history, the development of which can be traced back in various historical materials, is grounded in the conviction that diseases are unchanging. The majority of both historians and physicians, who in the

32 For more see Arrizabalaga, "Medical Responses," 36-7; French and Arrizabalaga, "Coping with the French Disease," passim.

33 Arrizabalaga et al., *The Great Pox*, 8.

34 For more on these bibliographies see subsection 3.1. of this work.

35 Gallus, *Bibliotheca medica*, 456.

36 Starting in the second decade of the 16th century, many printers began publishing a series of works devoted specifically to the French disease, but it does not appear that they also included consilia. Unfortunately, in his bibliography, Schenck does not mention in which of the published anthologies the relevant author appeared.

37 Lindenius, *De scriptis medicis*, 527-8.

38 Concerning the ontology of early modern diseases in general see Eckart and Jütte, M*edizingeschichte*; Lindemann, *Medicine and Society*. For the historiography of works concerning the pox in detail see Arrizabalga et al., *The Great Pox*, 3-16. For a detailed treatment of the ontology of diseases see Stein, *Negotiating*, 3-14; McGough, *Gender, Sexuality*, 9-16.

past studied the history of the French disease, clung to its ahistoricalism and was supported in this by today's nosological concept, according to which each disease is a definable unit, differing from others etiologically, morphologically or symptomatically. The term *syphilis* originated in the 16th century and it is generally known that this name was first used by the above-mentioned Italian physician Girolamo Fracastoro (1478-1553) in his poem "Syfilis sive de morbo gallico libri tres" (Syfilis or three books about the French disease) in the year 1530.[39] This designation did not catch on very well in the early modern period, which is testified to by the fact that none of the selected physicians used this name for the disease in their consilia (but for one exception).[40] Nevertheless, the concept of today's venereal syphilis, upon which our perception of the disease is based, only began to form at the end of the 18th century, when the most common term today began to be used more.[41]

Only at the beginning of the 19th century did the most important discoveries of bacteriology bring the definitive identification of "syphilis venerea."[42] In 1905, the cause of this disease was discovered by zoologist Fritz Schaudinn (1871-1906) and physician Erich Hoffmann (1868-1959). At this time, it started to become secondary what external symptoms the patient had, or how he felt, since the specific identity of a disease depended solely upon the visibility of the pathogen. At the same time, these discoveries meant the definitive fall of the classical and thus even the early modern concept of identifying diseases. However, historians started to take into consideration the fact that the early modern understanding of suffering and its perception is incompatible with the contemporary concept of venereal syphilis, since about the 1980s. Today the awareness about this disease as a phenomenon subject to historical changeability is more widespread, but nevertheless still to a lesser extent than in the case of the plague, for example. For these briefly outlined reasons, in this work there is a preference to designate the disease in question as the French disease, lues or the great pox.

39 The poem was written as early as 1521 and three years later this name was used by the renowned Erasmus of Rotterdam as a synonym for the French disease in his work. For more see Quetel, *The History of Syphilis*, 67.

40 The most common names in the selected consilia besides "morbus gallicus" were also "lues venerea" or "lues gallica," "morbus neapolitanus," or "morbus hispanicus." For understandable reasons, the last designations were preferred by French physicians.

41 A commonly used term even today, "Morbus venereus," or venerial disease, was supposedly first used by Jacques de Béthencourt of Rouen in the year 1527. For more see Quetel, *The History of Syphilis*, 53-4.

42 For more see e.g. Porter, *The Greatest Benefit*, 452-5.

4.3 The French Disease in Consilia Literature of the 16th Century

One of the oldest consilia in which the French disease figures, is supposedly a preventative-treatment consilium already written for the ruler of Heidelberg by his personal physician Konrad Schellig in the year 1495.[43] As already stated, because of its long course and seemingly incessant new outbreak waves, "lues gallica" was bound to appear in consilia literature continuously. In the period to which this study is devoted, the pox was already endemically spread and notoriously well-known to the physicians whose collections have become the main topic of this work. Several of them were born before the outbreak of its epidemic stage, but nevertheless at the time, when they likely completed their studies of medicine and started to practise, the French disease already existed in its chronic form, its symptoms were (within the bounds of diagnostic possibilities) well-known and the two most important medicines, mercury and guaiacum, were being used for its treatment.

The study of the selected consilia offers a range of interesting questions to research. Is the fact that in the 16th century this disease was considerably widespread even in the highest social circles reflected in the number of consilia? Was this disease already viewed at that time as "morally defective," thus were physicians conspicuously more discreet regarding the personal information of patients in these consilia? Was it common to mention the manner in which the patient got infected? Do these consilia also address theoretical questions such as the origin of the disease, manner of transmission, or reason for repeated attacks? Does the fact that of the fifteen creators of consilia collections or anthologies in this probe, several were also the authors of independent treatises concerning the nature and treatment of the French disease manifest itself in the number of consilia or in the theoretical passages?[44]

43 For more Arrizabalaga et al., *The Great Pox,* 89.

44 The already mentioned bibliographer, Pascal Lecoq, in his *Bibliotheca* from the year 1590 under the subtitle "Scriptores de Lue Venerea," captured four names, whose bearers also appeared in connection with consilia: B. Victorius, R. Solenander, I. Fernelius and I. Montanus. For more see Gallus, *Bibliotheca medica,* 456-7. Physicians, whom the previously mentioned bibliographer Schenck cited as authoring independent treatises on the French disease and are also among the figures writing consilia, include: B. Victorius, H. Capivaccius, I. Montanus, I. Crato, I. Fernelius and R. Solenander, a total of six personages. For more see Schenckius, *Biblia iatrica,* passim. The last bibliographer, van der Linden, again only noted four physicians: B. Victorius, H. Capivaccius, I. Montanus and I. Crato, who were connected both with consilia literature and treatises concerning the French disease. Lindenius, *De scriptis medicis,*527-8.

Many more questions could be asked, but since the consilia on the French disease are only meant to clearly document the interesting information in consilia literature, the number of problems studied will be limited. Naturally, we will be interested in the number of consilia for syphilis patients in each individual collection and the detail of the indications of patients, such as their social status or names. In the area of pharmacology, our attention will focus on only the two most important medicines for the French disease – guaiacum and mercury. One formula can be composed of even twenty items and many formulas can be found in a single consilium, so the use of other treatment ingredients will only be mentioned in passing.[45] In addition to these basic factors, certain specific interesting points, which could complete the known facts known up until now regarding communication, mutual collaboration between physicians and their private life and relationships with patients, will be pointed out. One of the consilia will be presented with its complete text.

Before we focus on the collections and anthologies examined, several important observations which influence the results of every study concerning any historical disease need to be taken into account. Firstly, we must not forget that in the early modern period, just as in the Middle Ages, the primary diagnostic methods involved examining the pulse and urine, evaluating subjective perceptions in the fluctuations of temperature and external symptoms noted through observation.[46] Although the external symptoms of the French disease may appear quite conclusive to us compared with other diseases, this impression is deceptive. No uniform classification of diseases existed and lues was not thoroughly differentiated from other venereal or dermal diseases of a different origin.[47] In the case of consilia, the physician moreover often had to depend solely on the symptoms put down in writing, which a colleague sent him. The experience level and reliability of the colleague concerned was also not necessarily of high standard. For these reasons as well, it is evident why historians of medicine today look to the possibilities of retrospective diagnosis.[48] Although it would perhaps be

45 For more about the number of ingredients, see e.g. Divišová, "Problematika syfilis," 107-9.

46 Concerning the main diagnostic methods generally see e.g. Nicolson, "The Art of Diagnosis," 801-18, et al. In greater detail, see e.g. Stolberg, *Die Harnschau.*

47 Even in the 18th century, it was not yet possible to resolve the long-lasting dispute of whether gonorrhea was the initial phase of syphilis. For more see e.g. Porter, *The Gratest Benefit,* 280-1; Quetel, *The History of Syphilis,* 82-3; Brandt, "Sexually Transmitted Diseases," 567-8.

48 On retrospective diagnosis see Cunningham, "Identifying Diseases in the Past;" Arrizabalaga, "Problematizing Retrospective Diagnosis; " Černý, "Problém retrospektivní diagnostiky;" Karenberg, "Retrospective Diagnosis; " Lindemann, *Medicine and Society,* 31-2.

wrong to reject it absolutely, it evidently cannot deliver reliable results. It has already been proven many times to be susceptible to new trends and fashionable diseases, and should be approached with great caution.[49] When assessing the diagnoses in the selected consilia, one should fully respect the contemporary medical discourse, the opinion of the physician and his diagnosis, regardless of how suspect it may seem to us. For this reason, we will only focus on consilia which include the French disease as the primary issue in their titles. Besides consilia, where the physician did not classify this disease as lues despite seemingly clear symptoms of the pox, we will not (save for several justified exceptions) analyze in detail any consilia where the pox is only mentioned in the text, e.g. in the anamnesis of the patient or as a "secondary issue" to more important health problems.

4.4 Advice for Syphilis Patients from Selected Authors

Although syphilis was a common disease in the upper echelons of society, the consilia for syphilitics were not included in every collection. They do not figure at all in the works of three of the selected physicians. For understandable reasons, we find no consilia concerning this disease from Johannes Matthaeus, whose only recipient of consilia care suffered from gout. Surprisingly however, we also learn nothing from Jean Fernel, who was not only the author of a new medical system, but also the author of a groundbreaking treatise about this disease. Although the index of his collection of 79 consilia mentions a consilium titled "Lues venerea cum aliis symptomatis," it cannot be found here or in any other republication.[50] The third physician and at the same time editor of the collection, where no patient afflicted by the French disease appears, was Diomedes Cornarius. It is unlikely that he did not encounter this disease, but rather did not include it for some other reason. Although there are relatively few consilia for syphilis patients from the remaining authors, it is not possible to focus on the content and form of each individual consilia separately. For authors where consilia for the treatment of the French disease are more frequent, only the most important ideas and common points will be highlighted and summarized, while some individual consilia will be examined in greater depth.

49 For a positive evaluation of retrospective diagnosis see Stolberg, *Homo patiens*, 215-6.

50 Fernellius, *Consiliorum medicinalium liber*, 1582; Fernellius, *Consiliorum liber*, 1585; Fernelius, *Consiliorum medicinalium liber*, 1589; Fernelius, *Consiliorum medicinalium liber*, 1597.

From among the consilia of the oldest selected physician, Paduan professor Benedetto Vettori, only one is dedicated to the treatment of the French disease. Its recipient was a representative of the ecclesiastical class, who in addition to the great pox also suffered from some form of vertigo, a hernia and vision problems.[51] "Treatment of the French disease by means of medications" (Curatio morbi gallici per medicinas) began traditionally with purging and continued with detailed treatment instructions with a daily schedule and formulas for individual preparations. Fundamental emphasis was put on the regimen.[52] Vettori favored simplicia, meaning common plant ingredients. He also recommended the already tried and tested guaiacum, but only if the previous medicaments did not work. He strongly warned patients against the use of mercury: "I advise the gentleman not to undergo the mercury coating because of the damages that could easily occur, ..." He however only devoted one single sentence in the entire instructions to both of the primary medicaments.[53] For treatment of the pox he also recommended baths with an infusion of herbs and the final two pages were dedicated to the treatment of the patient's other ailments.[54]

According to the index of diseases, there are no other consilia in the collection on the treatment of the pox. Nevertheless, the first consilium of the collection is a case where lues eventually appears in the patient's more detailed anamnesis. Because precisely this consilium concerns an important, identifiable figure and can be dated, it will be the first exception that breaks the resolution to ignore such consilia. The consilium was written for Bishop of Trient, Cardinal Bernard von Cles, Chancellor to Emperor Ferdinand I.[55] The consilium written four years before his death concerned "various bodily problems, especially of the brain and things related to the affliction of the brain."[56] In the consilium (33 standard pages long according to contemporary measures), the Paduan physicians, since

51 Victorius, *Medicinalia consilia,* 1556, 284v. Cons. XXXIX.

52 Ibid., 284v.-6r. "Curatio morbi gallici" is based on the selection of the right foods, and no conceivable component of diet or beverages was omitted: meat, fruit, vegetables, eggs, oils, wine, milk, etc. Due to this, the consilium is long by today's standards at 37 standard pages.

53 Ibid., 287v. "... consulo, ut non submittatur inunctioni ex mercurio propter nocumenta, quae ... facile contingere possunt, cum autem devenire ad potum decoctionis aquae ligni Guaiacani ..., non possum vituperare, sed summe laudare."

54 Ibid., 287v.-8r.

55 Bernardus Clesius (d. 30.7.1539), see di Rill, Dizionario Biografico degli Italiani, 26., 1982, https://www.treccani.it/enciclopedia/bernardo-cles_%28Dizionario-Biografico%29/

56 Victorius, *Medicinalia consilia,* 1556, 5r. Cons. I. "Pro ... Bernardo Clesio, ... Cardinali Ampliss. et Tridentinorum Episcopo. Ad varias corporis ... affectiones." The consilium was written at the Padua Faculty of Medicine on September 24th 1535.

this time they were the conclusions of an actual meeting, first engaged in a thorough analysis of the poor physical constitution of the patient.[57] Near the end of the detailed commentary an inconspicuous note that requires no explanation appears: "At the age of 23 years ... fortune played an unkind trick on him, he caught the French disease."[58] A description of the symptoms follows – cachexia, headaches, disintegration of the palate etc.[59] The physicians stated that the patient had been treated with mercury in previous years, and warned him of the threat of paralysis. They saw the remedy in the correct regimen rather than medications.[60] Despite this, they proposed several preparations of simplicia and a potion made of guaiacum. They mentioned the cardinal's personal physician, Hieronymus Drogo of Parma, with high praise. It is highly probable that he requested the consilium from the Paduan professors.[61] In the remaining five chapters, the council dealt with other manifestations of the patient's disease.[62] The remains of the cardinal have not undergone a modern paleopathological examination, so it is not possible to confirm whether he actually suffered from the said disease. However, thanks to this consilium, we can say that a suspicion exists that the future cardinal caught a venereal disease during his studies of law in Bologna and because of it died.

In the collection of another important Paduan professor, Giovanni Battista da Monte (Montanus) one can find "morbus gallicus" in the subtitles of 24 consilia. The consilia in the publications researched were organized into blocks according to the concerned problems. The French disease was given a separate section, but also appeared in other consilia as a secondary problem to another disease.[63] Da Monte's consilia are particular in that a large part were created in hospitals (or in the households of patients) as a record of an instruction presentation, so their texts are interlaced with a large number of rhetorical questions, which the lecturer immediately answers themself.[64]

57 Ibid., 5r.-6v. Intemperies denoted a disruption of the balance of fluids in the body.

58 Ibid., 6v. "Anno igitur 23. aetatis suae D.V. Reverendissima, contumaci favente fortuna, Gallica affectione corripitur."

59 Ibid., 7r.-8v.

60 Ibid., 9v.-10r.

61 Ibid., 15v.-19r.

62 Ibid., 19r.-22v.

63 Montanus, *Consultationum medicarum opus.* Similarly, even in consilia other than of the French disease, we find the treating of related diseases, the treatment of which is sometimes considered more important than treating the pox itself. E.g. 852, Cons. CCCLVII.

64 For more concerning the course of Montanus's instruction see Bylebyl, "The Manifest and the Hidden in the Renaissance Clinic," 40-60.

One of the strongest common characteristics of consilia for syphilis patients is the vehement attacks against the use of mercury.[65] He warned his students against its effects in the following way:

> "... a physician ordered ointment made of cursed mercury and moreover in the wrong proportion. That is the greatest offense. I saw how a teaspoon in which mercury was left overnight was broken; such and so terrible is the strength of mercury. And the surgeon coated this man's entire face, arms up to the elbows and part of the shins. ... Previously, almost everything was coated in the course of treating the French disease. That caused what we see during the autopsies of those treated, that the substance of their brains is soaked in mercury. ... I have nothing to say concerning mercury and have never considered it anything but a poison ..."[66]

Da Monte supported his aversion to mercury with the affirmative opinions of classical physicians, especially of Galen, who, as opposed to representative of Arab medicine Avicenna, always completely rejected it.[67] Besides classical authorities, he also used the testimonies of his renowned contemporaries. "... from experience I have observed that there is nothing worse for the afflicted than to use... in the form of an ointment or smoking that which contains mercury. And I swear – and the noble Fracastoro was present – that from the mercury coating someone immediately fell into epilepsy and was just hardly saved."[68] Da Monte for this reason preferred an ointment made of Virginia creeper with additives from hydrocerussite, lead and deposits of other metals and lime.[69]

For evident reasons he was even more strongly against the internal administering of mercury.[70] He was especially against the mercury preparation

65 Montanus, *Consultationum medicarum opus,* e.g. 853-4, CCCCLVII. "... the patient was punished with many afflictions, which stem in part from the great pox, partially from the accursed use of mercury." Ibid, 817, CCCLVIII. "... to this they added a mercury ointment and that is the worst cause ..."

66 Ibid., 868.

67 Ibid., 838. "But in addition to experience, we have ... all Greeks knew the same and Galen never spoke of it otherwise than as a poison. ...As when Avicenna wanted to try mercury and the same as other Arabs, who were great alchemists, he openly explained all of its disadvantages and how it leads to paralysis ..."

68 Ibid., 838.

69 Ibid., 850-1, CCCLVI. Surprisingly, in this consilium he left out guaiacum.

70 Ibid., 869. "Wherefore Empiricists were to be expelled from the town even with their secret because they kill many people. They use a pill with mercury ...;" 876, Cons. CCCLXII. "Concerning someone, whose use of mercurium praecipitatum in the treatment of the great pox corroded

mercurius praecipitatus, behind the spread of which supposedly stood the renowned healer Leonardo Fioravanti.[71] Fioravanti was a representative of a wide and diverse group of healers, who played a much more significant role than university-educated physicians in its treatment at the beginning of the epidemic of French disease. Since after the outbreak of the new disease, healers quickly reacted with an offer of "guaranteed" medications, they filled somewhat of a care and treatment vacuum into which the sick fell because of the hesitation of doctors expertly disputing the classification of the new disease.[72] In later times, however, representatives of healers or "charlatans" did not actively participate in the treatment of the French disease in any way. Physicians, barber-surgeons and pharmacists assumed their role.[73]

Reproachful addresses, where da Monte criticized patients for their lifestyles by which they enabled the inception of a disease or made its treatment impossible, were no less frequent than his attacks on mercury.[74] The commentary naturally concerned the "six non-innate things" and the strongest reproaches were earned by patients from Poland and Germany. So we read that the patient "so erred in the six non-innate things that it is surprising that he is not already long dead," and furthermore "... he came across an infected person [woman] and caught the French disease, wanted treatment and used mercury."[75] An interesting commentary is found in a consilium for a noble Pole for the sake of whom a consilium was held right at da Monte's house in the year 1544.[76] According to da Monte, from among the external causes, the condition of the patient, in addition to the use of "accursed mercury," was primarily the fault of the air (one of the six non-innate things), which is in Poland "in the winter so cold that nails fly out with such strength that they kill people."[77] Da Monte commented that

his stomach." *Mercurius praecipitatus* is mercuric oxide. For more on its production and use see Priesner and Figala, *Alchemie. Lexikon*, 56.

71 For more about Leonardo Fioravanti and his medicine see Eamon, *The Professor of Secrets*, 300.

72 For more see Arrizabalaga et al., *The Great Pox*, 28-9, 253-8. The first university-educated physician, who used internally administered mercury pills, was the renowned Pietro Andrea Mattioli. For more see Quetel, *The History of Syphilis*, 61.

73 For more see Gentilcore, *Medical Charlatanism*, 197-8.

74 Montanus, *Consultationum medicarum opus*, 877. Cons. CCCLXVIII. "The causes that could have induced this attack were food and drink."; 854. CCCLVIII. "... externally the French disease was worsened by the wrong medicines and a poor lifestyle;" 853. Cons. CCCLVII. "The disease will not be cured ..., until the patient begins to live moderately ..." It is essential to note that the right regimen was the foundation of the balance of the fluids in the body.

75 Ibid., 112.

76 Ibid., 814, Cons. CCCXLVIII.

77 Ibid., 817.

he would require three days to completely list the patient's transgressions against the regimen.[78] The same criticism of an immoderate life also appears in the case of another patient from Poland, who the Paduan physicians managed to cure despite a disintegrated nose and throat.[79] Another patient from Germany was reproached for drunkenness and overeating, while at the same time da Monte also "lambasted" his physician because he bled him too much and prescribed him mercury.[80] In this consilium, da Monte held a longer explanation concerning the nature and manners of transmission of the concerned disease, which as stated above were not by far clearly designated. Da Monte never concealed that patients became infected through sexual intercourse.[81] In addition, here he mentioned transmission via breast milk.[82] Even here we find consideration of the discussed quality of the disease and transmission mechanism. He designated the effect of an occult quality, due to which lues is related to rabies, as the essence of the disease.[83] In connection with this, da Monte further stated that lues is nearly untreatable in cholerics, while he gave phlegmatics, sanguinics and melancholics a pretty good chance.[84]

It is worth mentioning consilia for a group of patients, where physicians were supposed to decide whether they really suffered from that unpleasant disease. Sometimes the diagnosis was evidently easy: "When I heard the description of the course and type of pain of this noble youth, the French disease seemed to me to be described and depicted as if I had it before my own eyes."[85] In several cases however, physicians could not agree.[86] One of these was a certain Jew in whose case da Monte came to a negative conclusion after a lengthy analysis of all symptoms. Although the described symptoms were identical to those of syphilitic patients, according to da Monte's assertion "all Hebrews are ... melancholics, have thick blood and cool

78 Ibid.

79 Ibid., 846-50, Cons. CCCLV.

80 Ibid., 857, Cons. CCCLX.

81 Ibid., 112, Cons. XLIIII. "... he enjoyed coitus immoderately and ... came upon an infected woman and caught the French disease ...;" 835, CCCLII. "... he lay with a woman infected with the French disease (cum infecta muliere) and caught boils on the genitals ...;" 844, "... he had intercourse with an infected woman;" 853, CCCLVII. "... he had that thing with an infected woman (cum contagiosa muliere);" 873, CCCLXVI. "... he enjoyed himself with a prostitute (cum scorto) and caught the French disease."

82 Ibid., 858.

83 Ibid., 858.

84 Ibid., 859.

85 Ibid., 844. Cons. CCCLIIII.

86 Ibid., 812, CCCLXVII.; 864-7, Cons. CCCLXII.; 871-3, Cons. CCCLXV.

livers, ... so the symptoms are deceptive ..."[87] The patient was subsequently treated for only catarrh and melancholy. It is important to note that for the same reasons other experts considered melancholics as especially susceptible to the French disease.[88] A consilium for the wife of a patient from Germany, who da Monte treated because of the French disease, delivered the same result for similar reasons.[89]

Worth mentioning is da Monte's explanation of the great pox, which appeared in several consilia. Here, da Monte touched upon all essential questions discussed in professional circles: what does the term "epidemic" mean in connection with the French disease, the theory of the aging and subsequent weakening of the disease and its origination in the army of Charles VIII.

> "... I believe that the French disease cannot be designated as epidemic because epidemic [diseases] have universal causes (as Galen says in the first book of "Epidemics"), either air or food and drink... many years have already passed since the time when this infection began, and I believe that it should already decline. ... In addition to this, we know that our forbearers observed that at that time nobody became infected otherwise than through contagion (*contagium*): that had a particular cause. We know that at that time, when the French King waged war near Naples, there were many Spaniards, who arrived from Calicut, there.[90] In those lands, infection is plentiful and because they [the Spaniards] had a good time with prostitutes, the prostitutes were infected through this intercourse and the infection finally arrived here because there were women and soldiers of all nations. And from historical cases (*ex historiis*) it is known, ... that it is not treated with anything else than only wood [guaiac], which was brought to us. However, whether to classify this disease its nature with those from poor constitution, those from continuous unwinding or poor temperament is the greatest difficulty."[91]

87 Ibid., 330-1, Cons. CXXXIII.

88 Arrizabalaga, "Medical Responses," 39.

89 Montanus, *Consultationum medicarum opus*, 861, Cons. CCCLXI.; 857, Cons. CCCLX. is for her husband.

90 Today the city of Kozhikode in southern India; da Monte certainly meant America.

91 Montanus, *Consultationum medicarum opus*, 835, CCCLII. "Concerning the French disease for a noble German N. Prumer." The consilium took place in Padua on June 11th 1542 in collaboration with a surgeon and several other physicians. Worth mentioning is the patient's detailed anamnesis, which even mentions the patient's childhood diseases, e.g. middle-ear infections. For more on manners of categorizing and classifying diseases see e.g. Černý, *Mor1480-1730*, 149-50.

After the brief survey of da Monte's opinions on this disease and its treatment, I will take the liberty of pointing out several details from two consilia. The first was selected because of the less common manner of treatment and the mention of da Monte's father. The patient was apparently very wealthy because before da Monte his treatment was also led (in addition to many other physicians) by Antonio Musa Brassavola, the personal physician to the Dukes of Ferrara and author of a valued treatise on the French disease.[92] Da Monte surprisingly recommended to this patient a thermal spring cure, which other physicians warned against, and only after the baths failed did he prescribe guaiacum. And while in other consilia for his syphillis patients he strictly forbade sex, he allowed this patient "because he had a wife, to have intercourse out of necessity, not for pleasure and limited movement [during it]."[93] Da Monte called insistently upon patients to follow his orders and treatment and used the case of his father as a cautionary tale of the insidiousness of the disease and neglect of treatment: "… that disease is cursed with various symptoms; if it is not treated correctly, it creates thousands of changes even after many years. [Montanus] mentioned his father, who did not want to believe that he had that disease because he had not touched any [woman] in many years. He did not use the designated medications and died of it."[94]

The final consilium from da Monte that will be mentioned was intended for a member of a famous family of condottier, Galeotto II. Pico della Mirandola, a relative of the renowned Humanist of the same name. Thanks to the dates given, we know that it was written less than five months before the patient's death.[95] After an analysis of his temperament, or physical constitution, he and his colleagues recommended that the patient especially tame his quick-tempered nature and limit the physical exertion connected to military life.[96] This and the subsequent advice concerned the "six non-innate things," meaning the regimen. Although da Monte appeared to put an end to the topic of eating with the words "… another list of foods is a thing so well known that I don't want to sing this same old song over and

92 Montanus, *Consultationum medicarum opus*, 856, Cons. CCCLIX.

93 Ibid., 857.

94 Ibid.

95 Ibid., 823, CCCLI. "The consilium, which shows the treatment of the French disease and almost all its unusual symptoms, especially cracks. Given to the noble Galeotto Pico Mirandola, in June of the year 1550. Translated from Italian by Hieronymus Donzellini." Galeotto II. Pico della Mirandola (d.20.11.1550, Paris).

96 Ibid., 825.

over again," he did not abandon this topic.[97] He considered it important to take into account the frequent stays of the patient in France and supplement his dietary advice focused on the specialties of French cuisine.[98] After instructions concerning the treatment of boils, purgation and prescriptions for catharsis, da Monte warned the patient against another attack of the French disease, which could be triggered by travel stress.[99] He did not fail to note the uniqueness and effectiveness of guaiac wood, "which is God's gift."[100] Formulas for the preparation and instructions on the use of medicaments made of guaiac and many other ingredients took up several pages.[101] At the end, da Monte warned against external manifestations of the disease, like spots, pustules and the loss of hair, which are "... [things] humiliating to see and very inopportune for a life in politics," and offered him many prescriptions that could help to eliminate these cosmetic problems.[102]

In the collection, or rather anthology of another Paduan professor, Vittore Trincavelli, one can find seven consilia for syphilis patients among the 76 consilia.[103] However, Trincavelli's colleagues, whose opinions were recorded separately, contributed to five of these consilia. If we understand these parts as separate consilia, the number of consilia for syphilis patients increases to seventeen. However, even on the other cases, Trincavelli could have collaborated with someone else, as evidenced by his words from the consilia under which only he himself is signed: "The issue about which we should speak is absolutely clear ... it is the French disease, a contracted contagion (ex contagio), and there is no reason to discuss this in length now ..."[104] In a theoretical analysis, Trincavelli focused in detail on the question of so-called putrefaction in the body (putredo), and furthermore instructions for catharsis and treatment.

> "When the body has been rid of those harmful wastes, it doesn't seem good to me to stop. It is necessary to proceed on to medicines, which experience has shown as effective in destroying this malignant plague and in altering the imbalance of humors that is the source (fomes) and

97 Ibid., 826-7.
98 Ibid., 829.
99 Ibid., 829-30.
100 Ibid., 830.
101 Ibid., 831-2.
102 Ibid., 832.
103 Trincavellius, *Consilia medica*.
104 Ibid., 689-91, Cons. CXX. Lues Gallica.

> foundation of that evil. They are especially these three [medicines] (I would omit mercury ointment because I cannot approve it in this case): decoction of guaiac wood, decoction of sarsaparilla root and decoction of the China root."[105]

No more-detailed instructions were provided, but Trincavelli's colleague likely addressed them in an unrecovered consilium.

On the other hand, in the consilium "Scabies and the French disease" (Scabies cum lue Gallica) Trincavelli followed the ideal composition of consilium: after the theoretical presentation and anamnesis, he put together a precise diet and medication treatment with procedures for the patient.[106] The somewhat confusing title of the consilium only documents the symptomatic nature of the early modern nosological system. Here, according to the following description, by scabies is meant a syphilitic rash. In the following consilia, two other colleagues from the faculty always appear. Trincavelli most often collaborated with Luigi Bellocato.[107] Other physicians: Bassiano Landi, Gabriele Falloppio, Girolamo Capivaccio and Antonio Fracanzani appear only once, and in two consilia, one of the participants in the consilia is not identified. We cannot say who recorded the consilia, but students cannot be ruled out. For most of these consilia, it is not clear whether the physicians consulted the cases in a hospital, in the homes of wealthy patients, or just formulated a response to a request for assistance that they received. It is worth noting that the majority of these consilia were more expert opinions regarding a problem than a detailed proposal for treatment.

Just like da Monte, physicians in one case were supposed to confirm or refute a diagnosis. In the consilium on which the physicians Capivaccio, Fracanzani and Trincavelli collaborated they were surprisingly in concord that the patient – a noble young man with a boil on his lower leg, joint pain and problems with memory – did not suffer from the great pox.[108] The results of another consilium, where Trincavelli, Bellocato and an unnamed physician

105 Ibid., 690. Both sarsaparilla and china also had perspiration-promoting effects and sometimes replaced guaiacum. The china root (China smilax) and sarsaparilla were supposedly first mentioned in connection with the treatment of the French disease by physician Niccolo Massa in the year 1532. Physicians concerned that they might neglect some part of the treatment, sometimes prescribed a decoction of all these new components together. For more see Quetel, *The History of Syphilis*, 63.

106 Trincavellius, *Consilia medica*, 678-82. Cons. CXV.

107 Ibid., Cons. IX., XLIII., XLV., CXXI.

108 Ibid., 614. Cons. XCV. Arthritis: ulcus in crure: oblivio.

were supposed to evaluate a cured patient, his fertility and suitability for marriage, are hardly so uniform.[109] At the very beginning, critical words were aimed at the patient's attending physician: "A young, twenty-eight year old man, whose physical condition I was unable to recognize from either what was written, or orally stated, is introduced..." According to other information, the patient completed treatments using guaiac twice, a treatment using mercury vapor once, and when joint pain appeared the third time, a decoction from guaiac was used again. Despite shortcomings in the anamnesis, an unnamed physician from the council expressed the opinion that the patient was cured, but nevertheless he did not recommend marriage due to concerns of a relapse of the disease and because of his infertility. The opinion of Bellocato was different: he did not consider the patient cured due to joint pain and physical decrepitude. To remedy this, he recommended treatment using guaiac and to strengthen the body, the drinking of milk "however human, goat's or cow's milk, not donkey's milk, it is too thin ..."[110] He agreed with the previous colleague on the patient's infertility and also rejected marriage because of the infectiousness of the patient. Trincavelli only agreed with this in part: "I believe that he should not get married because he is too weak. I believe that he cannot infect a woman because the disease is aged ..."[111] The lack of unity in the opinions of consultants testifies to the importance of the patient's attending physician, who had to process consilia and draw a conclusion from them.

Another of the consilia, requested for "headaches due to the French disease" (Hemicrania Gallica), turned out similarly. Besides Trincavelli, the physicians Luigi Bellocato and Bassianus Landus also participated in this.[112] In his consilium, Bellocato determined the temperament, anamnesis of the patient and following a description of symptoms, he gave a prognosis. He viewed the possibility of a cure optimistically as long as the strongest medicine – guaiac was used after purgation and diet.[113] The second physician, Landus, surprisingly concluded that it was not the French disease and recommended a lighter treatment.[114] Trincavelli's opinion, which was supposed to decide the disagreement of the colleagues, only appears at the very end.[115] Based on a detailed analysis of temperament, he concluded that

109 Ibid., 691, Cons. CXXI. French lues: Emaciation: Gonorrhea.

110 Ibid., 692.

111 Ibid., 693. "Lignum Indicum" denotes American guaiac wood.

112 Ibid., 25-9.

113 Ibid., 26.

114 Ibid., 27.

115 Ibid., 27.

the patient was really suffering from the French disease and recommended using a decoction of guaiac wood.[116] To which opinion the attending physician finally inclined, we will never know.

The most interesting case, where in addition to treatment physicians were also asked for an evaluation, is even dealt with in two rather convoluted consilia. Paduan professors were supposed to decide whether the patient was suffering from the pox, was poisoned or enchanted.[117] The sick lawyer from Ferrara set off on the journey to Padua in person, but "was for no reason overwhelmed by fear that he would die on the way and so returned home," so the counsellors worked only with the written description of the attending physician.[118] The first participant of the convened council, who was perhaps the well-known G. Falloppio (see below), presented a description of the symptoms (boils, gummata, memory loss etc.) and an overview of the previous treatment of the Ferrara and Milan physicians.[119] In the course of the detailed anamnesis, he also reported the finding of clean wool and other strange materials in the excrement of the patient, which aroused suspicion of the use of magic and because of which, monks were called for assistance.[120] This physician was hesitant with regards to magic, but was clear concerning the French disease:

> "... on the right in the stomach [is] a tumor, perhaps one could find something similar to wool inside it. But if you open up silkworms, there is silk in them: if you chop open spiders, you find threads in them. If therefore hair can grow on certain parts of the human body, perhaps even those fibers originated in the bowels. But I think rather that it is something ingested by the mouth. ... he entrusted himself [into the care] of Ferrara maidservants: perhaps the black, hard excrement was magic in which wool was used. He lives in a mountainous region, where witches (feminae

116 Ibid., 28

117 Ibid., 442. Cons. XLIII. "Melancholy related to the lower abdomen: French disease: tumor in the area of the right groin."

118 Ibid. pg. 443.

119 Ibid, pg. 443. "It is 25 years that he is afflicted by a difficult office and worries, ...which called up his passion; he became close with a servant and small short-lasting boils appeared on the genitals. Those nevertheless disappeared after he was cleaned, then they appeared again ... he retired to Milan, where a physician concluded that it is a French boil and cured him by cauterizing them. As soon as he returned to Ferrara, a headache appeared ..."

120 Ibid., "... in his excrement was found a white, clean wool ... someone suspected nefarious powers ... Also discovered was something similar to soil, black, oval, very foul-smelling, which he proclaimed to be a "tongue of a rook" here used by sorcerers. He called up several monks, who believed that they could cure him ..."

> magae) usually dwell, especially in our Mutino region ... Concerning the other problems ... he suffers from the French disease. He was namely very hedonistic and had a good time indiscriminately with everyone the servant brought in."[121]

In the instructions for treatment after catharsis, blood-letting and baths, he recommended formulas for various syrups and finally "if the lues were to gain in strength, I would use guaiacum."[122] Bellocati and Trincavelli essentially agreed with the opinion of the first physicians, and both recommended guaiacum in the treatment, but Trincavelli differed in the other ingredients because he considered the French disease treated and not very dangerous.[123] The same lawyer is also the subject of yet another consilium, which is likely just a second record of the same consultation.[124] Professors Falloppio, Bellocato and Trincavelli commented on this case, so the unnamed physician in the previous case was probably Falloppio.[125]

Another professor of the same faculty, Girolamo Capivaccio, who was also the author of a separate treatise on lues, has only two on this topic preserved among "his" 51 consilia.[126] Similarly to the previous representatives of this renowned medical school, besides Capivaccio, other physicians, evidently members of the convened faculty council, Girolamo Fabrici d' Acquapendente and the more specifically unknown N. Nigri, commented on one of the cases here as well.[127] Fabrici mentioned in the anamnesis that the patient fell ill about 14 years ago and seemed to have been cured with a concoction of guaiac.[128] Then he contracted gonorrhea, which he attempted to treat with sexual intercourse on the advice of a Jew. Symptoms, which caused a wave of disputes between his physicians about whether it is the pox, followed. Diagnosis was made more difficult by the fact that the wife of the patient and their small children were healthy. Fabrici reacted with

121 Ibid., 443-4.
122 Ibid., 445.
123 Ibid., 445-7.
124 Ibid., 453-55, Cons. XLV. Hypochondriatic melancholy: French disease: etc.
125 For more concerning instructors at the Padua Faculty of Medicine see Ongaro and Martellozzo Forin, "Girolamo Mercuriale e lo studio di Padua," 29-50.
126 This treatise on the French disease was published by I. Hartmann Bayer in the same volume as *Opera omnia* as a consilium. Capivaccius, *Opera omnia,* 811-23. Posterior quincti libri pars. De morbo gallico.
127 Ibid., 956. Cons. XIII. "On hypochondriatic melancholy with vertigo, insomnia, and remains of the French disease."
128 Ibid.

an expert explanation in which he inclined towards the opinion that the patient is suffering from the French disease and according to this, he then proposed treatment; surgical procedures (blood-letting, fonticulus), lighter purgation, "alexipharmaca" made of guaiac, sarsaparilla and other simplicia.[129] Fabrici's colleague N. Nigri pronounced: "I wouldn't say that the French disease has been almost eliminated despite the fact that he felt relief after the concoction, he is not completely cured. It is nothing new that he has a healthy wife and children: I have seen the same in many other cases, who had both boils as well as gummata."[130] Even Capivaccio inclined in agreement towards the opinion of his colleague. He saw the salvation of patients in the best possible quality of medications of which he above all recommended the decoction of guaiac.[131] The collaboration and uniformity of opinions were completely ideal.

Cappivaccio was the only author of the second consilium on the French disease. He started traditionally with a description of symptoms, such as boils on the penis and eyelid, rash, swelling of the shoulders, but the longest part of the entire consilium was the theoretical analysis of the nature of the great pox.[132] This section clearly shows Capivaccio's view of contagion theory in which he held the dogmatic Galenic theory.[133] The prognosis was positive for the patient, but Cappivaccio did not refrain from criticizing the previous physician of the patient.[134] He first prescribed catharsis, then a decoction and pills from senna. He rejected guaiacum because it was too strong. He recommended a very weak decoction of guaiac only for the compress for the boil on the eyelid and for the penis a decoction of sarsaparilla or adder oil. Thus, he concluded his instructions for treatment because all else "is common knowledge."[135]

The penultimate Italian physician was Antonio Maria Venusti and one can find only one consilium on "lues Gallica" among his 28 consilia. The patient was an unnamed sixty-year-old civil servant and Venusti evidently

129 Ibid., 957.
130 Ibid.
131 Ibid., 958.
132 Ibid., 971, Cons. XXVIII.
133 Ibid., 971. "When someone becomes infected with the French disease (lues venerea) during coitus, he doesn't get a disease, but a cause of a disease, since the French poison (virulentia gallica), which is a warm matter, ... the infection (contagium) is proven by the presence of heat: after all, where there is contagion, there is decay (putredo), where there is decay, there is warming up (caliditas) ..."
134 Ibid.
135 Ibid., 972.

respected the patient's attending physician, who asked him for a consilium, largely because he approved in advance any changes by this physician to his proposed treatment. He proclaimed of himself that "he isn't the type" to defend his opinion tooth and nail against a better option.[136] Venusti approached it all in great detail (the same as all other consilia).[137] In the opening analysis he mentioned the history of the disease and its type, followed by a detailed analysis of the patient's temperament.[138] Venusti repeatedly emphasized the contagious character of this disease, so according to him, it could even be transmitted by used clothing.[139] The consilium contains extensive theoretical passages, e.g. an analysis of differences between the sexes in the constitution of the physical temperamentum, types of symptoms or general manifestations of the relevant disease. Only after these, was it the turn of the specific manifestations in the patient.[140] He then covered the regimen and selection of medicines in the same broad manner. However, unusual ingredients or procedures did not appear in any of them.[141] Although in the conclusion of the consilium Venusti left open the possibility of other methods of treatment, thus even mercury (for which he recommended studying the works of his teachers Falloppio, Fracanzani and Massa), he unequivocally preferred guaiacum.[142] In conclusion, Venusti called upon the attending physician to inform him about his own opinion.[143]

The editor of the last of the Italian authors, Cristoforo Guarinoni, included 35 consilia on the treatment of lues in the collection. They excel not only in their number, but also in their length so we will pause at only several selected consilia or passages from them.[144] One of the most striking characteristics of these consilia is Guarinoni's refined language and numerous

136 Venustus, *Consilia Medica*, 137-43. Cons. IX. Pro Assessore Vallis Ananiae, Septuagenario. De Lue Gallica. Clesii. (Anania, today Nonstal in Tyrol). Even here however are found cases of "cured" pox, which weren't included, e.g. 13-6. Cons. Pro Martino Malpaga, cive Tridentino. De regimine vitae a Lue gallica curatae.
137 Ibid., 137.
138 Ibid., 138.
139 Ibid., 139.
140 Ibid., 140.
141 Ibid., 141-3.
142 Ibid., 142.
143 Ibid., 143. "Tu autem quid sentias, expecto."
144 Common among the consilia of C. Guarinoni are consilia that would according to today's norms be 40 standard pages in length, some even over one hundred standard pages, but naturally even the complete opposite appear.

theoretical-philosophical explanations, which occasionally caused him to stray from the original topic. The very first consilium on the treatment of lues is evidence of this. It is composed of an address intended for colleagues with whom he evidently worked on the case – he focused his attention exclusively on the anamnesis, while the patient evidently never lived to see the awaited instructions concerning treatment and formulas.[145] Worth mentioning is his sharp verbal attack on a colleague, who obviously had a different view of the disease and treatment: "... who wouldn't suspect [him] of longing for profit or fame, and certainly of the avarice to pronounce the greatness of his contributions before a powerful man? ... Do you at all doubt that they are the same symptoms, the same problems as at the start, but now much worse?"[146] Unfortunately, one cannot know whether it occurred in this way to the patient's attending physician, or one of the consultants, nevertheless, just about everyone lived to see reproaches from Guarinoni.

The problem that Guarinoni deals with in many of his consilia, and which we do not find in such abundance among the other authors, is epilepsy. He expressed the opinion that epilepsy originates from the French disease, or in connection with it, in nearly every consilium.[147] He saw one of its causes in luetic gummata, which he found in the autopsies that he personally conducted.[148] Epilepsy appeared even in a consilium for an unnamed young man, who was "healthy for two years" before the attack of the disease due to a mercury treatment.[149] Guarinoni considered this phenomenon as common and explained it at length with the existence of a tinder (fomes), which a disease weakened by the correct treatment and regimen leaves in the body and which can burst into flame again at any time.[150] He compared the latency of virus gallicum to rabies, but nevertheless not in quite the same way as da Monte did in his consilium. After a lengthy theoretical presentation about nerves, in which matter accumulates and the genesis of epilepsy occurs, he recommended a treatment of guaiac and sarsaparilla to the patient. He added a formula for a preservative (!) medicine to the instructions for the regimen at the end.[151]

145 Guarinonius, *Consilia medicinalia*, 17, Cons. XV. "On the treatment of the French disease."

146 Ibid.

147 Epilepsy appears in fifteen consilia, one even bears the title "On epilepsy from the French disease." See below.

148 Guarinonius, *Consilia medicinalia*, 18, Cons. XV.

149 Ibid., 18, Cons. XVI. "On epilepsy from the French disease."

150 Ibid. For more see e.g. Nutton, *The Reception of Fracastoro's Theory*, 200; Černý, "Mezi Fracastorem, Fernelem a Helmontem," 29.

151 Guarinonius, *Consilia medicinalia*, 18-9, Cons. XVI.

Guarinoni devoted greater attention than the other compared authors of consilia to astral influences on the development of disease. Besides the theory of epilepsy and treatment, he extensively addressed the astral influences in for example a consilium for a certain forty-year-old.[152] "I cannot pass over in silence the fact that when the moon wanes, problems escalate ... for the first time when the moon enters Aquarius and is close to its eclipse and rises in conjunction with Saturn, and for the second time when it is near the end of Scorpio with opposition to Mars ... "[153] He also applied his knowledge of astrology to another case in the course of which he took part in a meeting of a council composed of renowned physicians.[154] Guarinoni here (untypically for him) recorded in detail the psychological manifestations of the disease (or perhaps the consequences of previous treatment) of the 45-year-old patient afflicted by the pox for four years: "... he suffered cramps and neglected to care for himself several days and with a laugh accepted everything, even that which caused him the worst pain, ... full of fear ... he couldn't calm himself down or sit without immediately jumping up, looking around ... suspicious and who approached him, he attacked and immediately called them back and he swore at them ..."[155] After a theoretical analysis of all the usual components, filled with numerous citations from Galen and Hippocrates, Guarinoni addressed the influences of planetary conjunctions.[156] In the proposed treatment, he did not express himself entirely negatively towards mercury, but nevertheless he preferred the pleonastic extolled guaiacum. In addition to formulas for the preparation of medications, the effects of which as he proclaimed he had tried, he expanded his offering with the formulas of various other physicians and even recommended the use of amulets.[157]

The next consilium is evidently a continuation of the previous one. This time however, we learn at least some of the names of the consultants; Guarinoni was joined by the emperor's personal physician G. Alessandrini,

152 Ibid., 27, Cons. XXVIII. "On the French disease with many problems." Because of pain in the joints, there follows an analysis of the nature of rheumatism with numerous citations from Galen, analysis of the temperament of the patient, symptoms and analysis of the nature of apoplexy, 29. In connection with melancholy, a sirup, "... which was concocted by the Veronese Montanus" is recommended for its elimination

153 Ibid.

154 Ibid., 32-4, Cons. XXIX. De morbo gallico.

155 Ibid., 33.

156 Ibid., 37. "Unde non exiguum argumentum est, quo in venerea lue vis huius morbi posita est, Scorpione in naturalia apprime valente, ut planetis in eo versantibus semper malum venereum efferascere observatum Astrologis est..."

157 Ibid., 38.

professors of the faculty of medicine G. Capivaccio and G. Mercuriale, "and others."[158] After the anamnesis, Guarinoni addressed all three of the patient's problems: cachexia, epileptic seizures, and melancholy. One of the colleagues however refused to recognize the connection between these problems and the pox, so Guarinoni's consilium was transformed into a treatise on the nature of the origination of epilepsy, melancholy, and their connection with lues. He supported his deliberations with many examples and analysis of the patient's symptoms and temperament, and again noted the astrological influences.[159] For the treatment, he recommended in addition to catharsis, any medications, composed primarily of simplicia and guaiac. Colleagues however proposed substituting baths for guaiacum, against which Guarinoni strenuously protested in vain.[160] He made positive mentions of the influence of amulets and – somewhat skeptically – even concerning incantations. "One should not look down upon even amulets, like the stone called "cornolus," like the root of the peony and others. I wouldn't speak of words although of them, authors say that they are powerful if they are whispered in the ear during a seizure."[161] The treatment did not end successfully, and the patient was in the end against Guarinoni's will ordered treatment at the Paduan spa, where (unnamed) physicians forced him to write to "friends, prominent men (ad Principes viros), that he is recovering." After his return home, he had a seizure, of which the attending physician "upon whom the fault would fall" accused a demon (cacodaemon) and summoned exorcists. Guarinoni, called by the patient himself, was present at the exorcism and apparently even the subsequent death and autopsy, which he commented upon: "... after opening the head an entire half of the brain was filled with water and in the middle of all of the rot were three bodies as if of green rubber ..."[162] It is very likely that even the third consilium is connected with this case.[163] In it, Guarinoni informed one of the participants in the previous colloquium, Giulio Alessandrini, concerning the catastrophic results of the treatment of the patient at the spa in Padua. Guarinoni wrote this letter

158 Ibid., 39. XXX. Consilium de gallico cum Iul. Alexandrino, Hieron. Capivac., Hieron. Mercuriali et aliis pro ... etc.

159 Ibid., 39-42.

160 Ibid., 42-4. Guarinoni's opinion on the pointlessness of using baths for the treatment of the pox is captured in the collection once more, however as a "History;"for more see 49.

161 Ibid., 44. The verbatim translation would read "into the ears of the falling person," so this is again evidently an allusion to an attack of epilepsy.

162 Ibid.

163 Ibid., 44. Cons. XXXI. Clarissimo Viro Iulio Alexandrino S.C.M. Physico Primario. De symptomatibus convulsivis pro Illustrissimo N.

in Fossombrone in June of the year 1578 and emphasized in it that he was doing so at the explicit order of his masters, which he even had certified by a municipal physician. The connection between the above-mentioned consilia is very probable, so professors Capivacco and Mercuriale most of all bear responsibility for the unsuccessful treatment and death of the patient.[164]

Multiple consilia written for one patient were not an exception.[165] In one of these, in addition to an interesting formula for an alexipharmacum with guaiac, Guarinoni thus addressed the nature of the pox and its treatment: "Nevertheless, almost [all] better physicians have been forced to admit that its strength is unknown (occulta) to us ... And because when the nature of a disease is uncertain, we cannot select a medication through rational deliberation (certa ratione), but through a guaranteed experiment, we can deliver remarkable aid, and that is the guaiac potion ..."[166] In the subsequent consilia for the same patient, Guarinoni described detailed instructions for the preparation of the guaiac potion, a description of a "tent," which was used for sweating syphilis patients in home treatment, and in the dietary instructions forbade the patient sexual intercourse, although he mentioned that "... someone believes that it provides great relief [during attacks of the French disease], if the [ill patient] performs it with an untouched woman (integra mulier), and wishes to substantiate it with demonstration or proof (experiment).[167] It is a question, whether to interpret the term used by Guarinoni as "virgin," "healthy woman" or "virtuous woman," since in the history of sexually transmitted diseases all of these strange ideas have appeared. Sexual intercourse with a virgin was extolled by Spanish Humanist Juan Luis Vives (d.1540), and intercourse with a morally (but also physically) pure woman as a means of treatment was recommended by multiple physicians and it is likely that Guarinoni had their opinion in mind.[168]

The unsuccessful treatment of the above-mentioned patient and the necessity of defending his approach and exclusive use of guaiac and not mercury forced Guarinoni to write yet a third consilium.[169] In its conclusion, we learn

164 Ibid., 45. Because of the exact dating of the letter, it would probably be possible to even determine the identity of the patient.

165 Ibid., 283-4, Cons. CCLXIII. De morbo gallico. "Post luem morbi gallici nondum extinctam ..."; 286-288. Cons. CCLXV. De gallico morbo; 288-9. Cons. CCLXVI. Repetita novis auditoribus.

166 Ibid., 283.

167 Ibid., 287-8.

168 Arrizabalaga, "Medical Responses," 48-9. For more see Schleiner, "Infection and Cure through Women," 499-517; or (briefly only) Cunningham, *The Four Horsemen*, 255-6.

169 Guarinonius, *Consilia medicinalia*. 288. "... tantum dicam tam esse praeferendum caeteris remediis guaiacum, quam est certissimum omnium seculorum remedium, non paucorum, ut

that the patient died, however by the fault of the attending physician, who did not follow Guarinoni's instructions. Here, Guarinoni promised to address the problems further, but nevertheless the promised appendices were perhaps left out by the editor or could even have been detached and published as a separate consilium.[170] The possibility is strengthened by two "non-real" consilia-treatises on the treatment of the pox, which follow almost immediately.[171]

One cannot fail to draw attention to a consilium which is extraordinary in length, but most of all because of the patient. The introduction records Guarinoni's speech to the convened medical council: "We have gathered here, best men of the medical profession, and we were called here in order to find aid for the health of him, who is dearest not only to the nations subordinate to him, but also to the entire Christian world. And this especially applies to us, who to our joy live under his rule and great protection. ..."[172] The editor evidently left out the name of the patient, nevertheless readers could certainly deduce his identity, especially if, according to mentions in the text of the colloquium, it took place in Rome. The consilium continued in an ornate rhetorical style with extensive analyses of temperament, symptoms and treatment advice, accompanied by various digressions. The primary means of treatment was again to be guaiacum, the effectiveness of which Guarinoni swore by, despite his previous failed treatment of a patient. In the optimistic prognosis, he also mentioned the patient's (unnamed) brother, who apparently suffered from the same disease.[173] It is noteworthy that in this consilium Guarinoni used the name of the disease, which only became commonly used between the end of the 18th and beginning of the 19th centuries – syphilis. The following consilium on the French disease is evidently connected with the previous case.[174] It is a non-real consilium, since here Guarinoni defends the decisions and treatment approach of a five-member medical team. From his words we can gather that this group of physicians had apparently cared for the unnamed patient for a longer period of time and convened at least three times for a joint meeting. However, the agreed treatment approach was jeopardized by the calling up of another consultant upon whose head Guarinoni rained down criticism.[175]

caetera post ipsum prolata, quorum alia minus tuta sunt, ut hydrargyron, alia non ita efficacia ..."

170 Ibid., 289.

171 Ibid., Cons. CCLXIX. De gallico morbo.

172 Ibid., 387, CCCLXVI. "On the French disease for N." According to today's norms, the consilia is 30 standard pages in length.

173 Ibid., 391.

174 Ibid., 393, CCCLXVIII. De morbo gallico.

175 Ibid.

The large number of Guarinoni's consilia on the treatment of the pox makes the detailed examination of each one impossible. However, the selected examples have hopefully sufficiently documented Guarinoni's main opinions and his approaches to both treatment and structure of consilia. One characteristic trait of his unabbreviated consilia is pleonasm, an effort to demonstrate the depth of his knowledge. He vehemently defended the use of guaiac in treatment, but not without regard to the patient, when for example, he substituted guaiac for six-year-old theriac with an admixture of opium because the patient would be unable to stand the drastic diet connected with treatment using guaiac.[176] He even pronounced guaiacum, the effects of which he considered to be "occult," an *alexiteric*, meaning a panacea.[177] In order to augment its beneficial effects, he used not only supporting medications and preparations, but especially wine, which he was not afraid to recommend based on the results achieved by the Empiricists.[178] "Another way, which is not so generally approved of, but which I have seen cure many, is the use of wood [guaiac] from wine. This is used by the *empeirikoi,* and it is not surprising that the Empiricists can cure this disease in this way, after all we are not guided by reason (ratione), but rather by traditions adopted from others ..."[179] Guarinoni repeatedly blamed incorrect steps on the part of the patient or his attending physicians for any potential failure of treatment with guaiac.[180]

Patients whose physicians requested a consilium from Guarinoni were exclusively men. The collection contains only two consilia for women and in one a husband only requested a verdict as to whether it was a case of that unpleasant disease.[181] Just as with the other physicians, the collection of Guarinoni's consilia contains many diagnostic assessments.[182] In one case of the treatment of the pox, Guarinoni was himself the attending physician, who upon the patient's request forwarded his own consilium to

176 Ibid., 31, Cons. XXVIII. The older the medicine, the higher quality it was considered to be.

177 Ibid., 299, Cons. CCLXXVIII.; 394, Cons. CCCLXX. De gallico cum comitiali symptomate pro Illustrissimo, 395, "guaiac, tried over a long period and with many experiments, must be given preference before anything else ..."

178 Ibid., 324, Cons. CCCXV.; 153, Cons. CXXXVIII.; 291, Cons. CCLXXII.

179 Ibid., 292, Cons. CCLXXII. "Alia via est, non ita communiter probata, qua tamen vidi ego plures sanitati restututos, scilicet accepto eo ligno ex vino, hac *empirikoi* utuntur, nec mirum, quod empirici hunc morbum possint curare, nam nos quoque non tam ratione ulla, quam traditione ab aliis accepta dirigimur, ..."

180 Ibid., 280, Cons. CCLIIII.; 394. Cons. CCCLXX.

181 Ibid., 111, Cons. XCVI.; 612, Cons. DXXV.

182 Ibid., 82, Cons. LXIX.; 300, CCLXXIX.; 616, Cons. DXXVIII.; 623, Cons. DXXXV.

an unnamed colleague, whom he asked to confirm his course of action.[183] Several consilia could be classified as "epistolae medicinales" due to the fact that they were sent in the form of a letter and do not contain specific instructions for treatment.[184] And even in this collection, there are consilia which were not classified with those for syphilis patients because mentions concerning the patient's pox appeared in the anamnesis as a secondary issue. As an example, one can give a consilium for a prefect of the imperial guards in whose successful treatment besides guaiac, mercury was used internally which was extraordinarily rare.[185] However, here Guarinoni said of mercury that he did not like to use "such evil" internally, and he expressed moderate appreciation of mercury only for the treatment of less serious forms of scabies.[186]

We can now compare the refined language and somewhat lengthiness of Guarinoni's consilia with the work of his friend, the oldest of the selected physicians from North of the Alps, Johannes Crato von Krafftheim. Although Crato wrote a separate treatise on the French disease and an impressive seven anthologies of consilia were published under his name, only two consilia concerning the disease in question can be found among them. The first consilium essentially is only comprised of the treatment part, and we learn nothing about the patient himself, his anamnesis, or his temperament.[187] In treatment, Crato unequivocally preferred guaiacum and gave detailed instructions for the preparation of a decoction with instructions concerning its administering. Finally, he recommended supplementing guaiacum with purgatives and other preparations, for example a potion made of agaricum and senna. He also placed great emphasis on the quality of the herbs employed, fresh and dried in the shade.[188] In addition to the medications used internally , he also prescribed an ointment, the main ingredient of which was however Venetian soap, not mercury.[189] Regimen instructions, to which other physicians devoted dozens of pages, are comprised of a single sentence: "During the course of the entire treatment, he should avoid love

183 Ibid., 61. Cons. XLII. "Most noble sir, requested directly by the patient, I will briefly discuss his treatment with you."

184 Ibid., 394, Cons. CCCLXIX. De Gallico.

185 Ibid., 724, Cons. DCIIII.

186 Ibid., 384. Cons. CCCLXV.

187 Crato, *Consilorum liber quintus*, 254, Cons. XXXVIII. In morbo Gallico, pro quodam Nobili viro.

188 Ibid., 255. The mentioned prescription is composed of 27 herbal ingredients.

189 Ibid., 257.

and wine, stay away from [fresh] air as much as possible, not let in any night air at all and live as balanced a life as possible."[190]

Crato's second consilia on the treatment of the French disease also lacks any introductory history of the patient or disease, and in fact should not be counted among consilia for syphilis patients because above all it is a set of instructions for the right regimen for an already cured man.[191] The reason for maintaining the right regimen even many days after completion of the treatment according to physicians was the tenacity of the disease, which usually returned after no matter how small an excess and "changes into other and other forms."[192] An extensive list follows of the right and dangerous types of food, a recommendation of purgation with formulas for laxatives and the prescription of regular venesections.[193] Besides a strengthening medicine, the main component of which was theriac, he also recommended avoidance of coitus (especially after food and strong wine).[194] At the end of the consilium, in addition to instructions on the removal of pustules and macules, we find a rejection of treatment using mercury: "I wouldn't want to resort to medications made of mercuria and vaporization, which the inexperienced do not hesitate to use immediately."[195]

Even here, one cannot separate the volume compiled by L. Scholz from Crato's consilia, especially since the only two consilia on the French disease in this anthology are reprints of Crato's works. In the case of the first of these, titled "Consilium ... De morbo Gallico," is included Crato's separate treatise "De morbo gallico libellus" (Book about the French disease) and the second consilium is again identical to the above-mentioned consilium from the fifth volume.[196] The minimal number of consilia for syphilis patients among such a large number of consilia and their authors is surprising, but as has already been shown, the inclusion of consilia into print could have really just been a matter of chance and so that is what we will consider here.

190 Ibid.

191 Crato, *Consiliorum liber sextus,* 641, Cons. XCVI. For the remains and blisters of the French disease for a certain noble sir.

192 Ibid.

193 Ibid., 641-2. The foods that the patient should avoid include all "vestigial" meats, such as fish, especially carp, then pork, mutton and poultry living by water, such as e.g. geese; furthermore, fish prepared with butter, milk and all cheese foods.

194 Ibid., 645.

195 Ibid., 646.

196 Scholzius, *Consiliorum medicinalium liber,* 1042, Cons. CCCLXXXI.; 1056-7, Cons. CCCLXXXII. In morbo Gallico, pro quodam Nobili viro.

Only a single consilium on the French disease has been preserved in the collection of 136 consilia of Reiner Solenander.[197] The recipient was only a burgher and contacted Solenander, while the latter was working as a spa physician.[198] From the notes in the consilium, it is evident that they were in personal contact, but that at the time of the writing of this consilia, the patient was no longer staying in Italy. He suffered a second attack of the French disease and had been previously treated countless times with both guaiac and mercury, which according to Solenander, gave him "no fewer disadvantages than the disease itself." Solenander left out the usual purgation or catharsis of the body and recommended treatment at the spa, which according to the name were the renowned springs in Aachen.[199] This recommendation was accompanied by precise instructions concerning the length of the stay at the spa and a special drinking regimen. Besides this, Solenander placed an emphasis on regular evacuation and the right diet. He surprisingly rejected medications: "I would consider any other medicines that are swallowed to be superfluous in this case."[200] Several other pieces of advice concerned beverages, food and rest after the spa stay, and the physician did not express himself concerning many other things in writing since as he mentioned, he told them to the patient in person.[201] Despite this, he furthermore gives a formula for a decoction of guaiac or sarsaparilla and instructions for the length of use.[202] Mercury was recommended in a formula for an ointment for any possible rashes on the prepuce.

Even in the case of Solenander, a consilium-letter appears in which the diagnosis of the French disease was disputable. The young man, who contacted the physician because of concerns about the great pox, was very close to Solenander, as one can infer from both the style of communication and the amount of personal information about himself that he shared with Solenander.[203] Although a formula and instructions for a regimen appear here, a large part of the consilium is comprised of a private letter, where the

197 Solenander, *Consiliorum medicinalium sectiones*, 221, Cons. III. "For the excellent man Peter Budet, who is for a second time suffering from the French disease ..."

198 The consilium was written on July 17th 1574 at the spa in Lucca.

199 Ibid., 221-2.

200 Ibid., 222.

201 Ibid., 222-3.

202 Ibid., 223.

203 Ibid., 494, Cons. XVII. "... I was busy writing letters to patients and also partially getting ready for a trip – I am departing to see Mr. ... when I received your letter, ... full of lamentations ..."

physician tried in particular to encourage the youth from the psychological point of view.

> "Good God, how great is the strength of the spirit, when it rashly anticipates and listens not to any invitations of reason! ... be it any disease, be the infection ever so great and may it have put down, as it seems to you, any deep roots, it certainly is not that due to which you torment yourself. The disease of the spirit [in you] is already long worse than the malady of the body and that can cause much greater damage to your health. He, who asks that in a healthy body there be a healthy spirit, has the best attitude towards health. And so I beseech you on your health to fortify your spirit with reason ..."[204]

Solenander also invited the "founder of psychiatry," J. Weyer, who agreed that the young man yielded too easily to his notions, to assist.[205] At the end, Solenander expressed the concern that the youth in desperation could entrust his care "into the hands of some "agyrta" or roving charlatan, who "lacking knowledge of things and unaware of all bodily functions" would treat him with some sort of trickery. Unfortunately, not even here do we get the opportunity to confirm the correctness of the physician's diagnosis and learn how the case continued.

Among the 80 consilia, letters and observations of Guarinoni's contemporary, the German physician Johannes Wittich, we find only one with the title "On terminating the French disease (lues venerea) and other symptoms terrible to the sight, with the overall purgation of the body and a concoction of guaiac wood, of a certain noble count, composed and written by the sirs Johann Schröter and Johann Wittich."[206] This consilium includes three separate parts, or rather letters upon which besides Wittich, Jena professor J. Schröter collaborated. The first, longest part describes the instructions for the treatment of the disease concerned from J. Wittich.[207] Any information concerning the high status of the patient have been left out, and the consilium

204 Ibid.
205 Ibid., 497-8. "I haven't been at court in almost three weeks ... Doctor Wierus is filling in for me at court with respect to my duties. When he received your letter for me, he opened and read it. And so he added his opinion, which I am sending along with my own." 498. "Your messenger arrived yesterday around breakfast, I will send him back as soon as possible at three in the afternoon..."
206 Wittichius, *Medicorum consilia*, 541-58, Cons. LXXIIII.
207 Ibid., 54-2. "Curationis initium fiat ab hoc clystere A ..."

is comprised exclusively of formulas for various procedures (enema) and medicaments (formulas for decoction of guaiac, ointment, plaster, etc.) with precise instructions regarding their preparation and use.[208] Some of the Latin formulas also added instructions on how to call the preparation in German.[209] Mercury appeared twice in the formulas, but always only as a component of laxatives.[210] A "Victus ratio," meaning similarly detailed instructions for a regimen, especially food, drink and air, follows.[211]

The next part of the consilium for the same person consists of a letter from J. Schröter, who was evidently also a consultant.[212] Schröter wrote Wittich, who was related to him, that the man intends to marry and "... because of the completion of the man's treatment, it is necessary to share some essential things, which I cannot commit to paper. I will postpone my other affairs and will be happy to visit the man next week in order to together successfully complete the treatment ... together we will agree and prescribe something so that later any remnants of the evil will not spread and so that the contagion (contagium) could not appear on the children."[213] The third part of the consilium consists of a letter from Wittich to Schröter, but it is not a response to the above-mentioned letter from Schröter. The subject is the health of "count N. senior," who caused himself serious problems because "... he seriously erred in his regimen, when together with other courtiers he gave himself over to immoderate drinking of wine ..."[214] It further gives twelve formulas for "boils and cracks on the palms for the same count from Master Wittich and for luetic bumps on the penis."[215] It is not clear, whether it was about the same syphilis patient as the first part of the "consilium," or these formulas and instructions were part of another consilium.

208 Ibid., 543-4, "Postea sequenti die tribus horis ante prandium sumat hunc bolum ...;" 544-545, "Tertio hanc potionem usurpabit ...; 545, "... postea ad ligni decoctum accedat ..."

209 Ibid., 546-7. "... Signetur Morsellen nach dem schweis ... Sumat unum morsulum, ubi a sudore surrexit, hora una ante cibum. Signetur Leberstenglein ... Linimentum ... Signetur Sälblein zum leibe ..."

210 Ibid., 541; 547.

211 Ibid., 547-50. Wittich especially recommended the meat of young animals, poultry, and even song birds, to completely avoid milk; among beverages he only recommended fresh beer.

212 Ibid., 550.

213 Ibid., 550-1.

214 Ibid., 552.

215 Ibid., 552-8. "Ad serpigines et fissuras manuum pro eodem comite remedia a M. Wittichio ordinata; Ad tubercula penis a lue venerea; potio; Clysteres; rotulae praeservantes, morsuli, aqua, electuarium, ..." etc.

Among the 219 consilia of the last of the selected German physicians, Thomas Mermann, only one on lues is found, and that in the part devoted to problems "external, dermal and joint pain." The patient was a nobleman with the title of baron, and both the address and closing formula of the sent consilium hint that it was intended for Mermann's colleague, apparently the patient's attending physician.[216] This consilium is very brief and because of the fact that it does not deliver any specific proposals for treatment or a course of action, it should rather bear the designation of "epistola medicinalis." Concerning the patient, it only reports that he underwent balneological treatment. Mermann vehemently criticized the failure to follow the strict diet, since "he himself cannot remember anyone, who was properly cured of this disease, who had not felt hunger and endured it patiently."[217] Furthermore, he informed his colleague that in the local hospital he had seen syphilis patients successfully cured by "hydrargyrum praecipitatum" administered internally, but he nevertheless did not recommend "this evil" to the patient.[218] At the end he just asked the colleague to share the results of the treatment. However, on the copyright page of this "consilium" is printed information, which the editor a half century later considered valid and important: "N[ota]B[ene]. Who has not felt hunger in the course of the sweat cure of the French disease, will not be cured. Internally administered "hydrargyrum praecipitatum" treats the French disease."[219] As can be seen, at the time of the publication of Mermann's consilia, they looked entirely differently upon internal treatment with mercury.

French consilia literature is represented only by Guillaume de Baillou (Ballonius). In his first book, we apparently do not encounter any consilium on the pox, and from among the venereal diseases, only gonorrhea appears in the index.[220] Nevertheless, this one case of "gonorrhea" will however be briefly mentioned and will thus join the other exceptions. According to de Baillou, the unnamed patient was infected with gonorrhea, which turned into the Spanish disease (lues Hispanica) and with this he infected his pregnant wife. Their child, to the surprise of the physician, was born healthy, but "not long did that innocent scion bear the mark of the father's stain with

216 Mermannus, *Consultationes*, Liber VII. De malis externis et cutaneis, nec non articulorum doloribus; 501, Cons. XVIII. "The French boil."

217 Ibid.

218 Ibid., "Vidi hic in nosocomio malignitatem virulentiae istius hydrargyro praecipitato feliciter expugnatam per os assumpto."

219 Ibid.

220 Ballonius, *Consiliorum liber primus*, 464. Cons. XCII. De Gonorrhoea virulenta.

impunity…" After two months, on the entire body did appear "assured proof of the Spanish scabies" (scabies Hispanica).[221] In those times, physicians recommended discontinuing breastfeeding due to treatment and thereafter feeding the child from a glass bottle. The mother was subsequently treated with a concoction of guaiac, sarsaparilla and various types of theriac and mithridate for protection against the great pox. However, the infant was to be coated with mercury.[222]

In the second volume of de Baillou's consilia, only a single one on the French disease appears.[223] Elsewhere common information about the patient were left out with the exceptions of gender and symptoms. Instead of beginning with an anamnesis, de Baillou started by recording the indecision of the participating physicians concerning the diagnosis.[224] This was followed by de Baillou's instructions on how to recognize actual luetic pustules, and then he extensively addressed three interesting questions: why the Neapolitan disease afflicts the genitalia, the bodies of the long bones and not their ends and how this is related to nerves and joint pain.[225] This developed into a long treatise reminiscent of a presentation at the conclusion of which, in connection with arthritis, caused by luetic poison, appeared a defense of treatment using mercury.[226] Other proposals of treatment also headed more towards the theoretical level than to the patient concerned.[227] De Baillou vaguely recommended a strict diet, and although he considered mercury to be a "panacea" (alexipharmacum), he did not recommend it to patients because "it affects the brain and nerves adversely."[228] In connection with its use, he mentioned the criticism of the Empiricists, who used it only for financial profit.[229] At the very end, he furiously defended the use of wine in the course of treatment, which even the editor emphatically noted in his closing "Annotationes," where he summarized de Baillou's main ideas.[230] Since neither precise formulas, nor instructions for a regimen appear anywhere in the entire consilium, it is a question, whether or not to call this rather theoretical treatise a real consilium.

221 Ibid.
222 Ibid.
223 Ballonius, *Consiliorum liber secundus*, 185-92, Cons. II. De lue venerea.; 192-3, Annotatio.
224 Ibid., 185.
225 Ibid., 185-8.
226 Ibid., 188.
227 Ibid.,189.
228 Ibid., 190-1.
229 Ibid., 191.
230 Ibid., 192.

Another consilium for a syphilis patient appeared in the third volume of consilia, published with a quite large time delay after the first two.[231] Concerning the patient, de Baillou only mentioned that he exhibits many symptoms of incipient pox, and in order for him to be cured, he must use the prescribed medicines and follow the appropriate regimen.[232] This is followed by a recommendation concerning food, next a formula for an enema, instructions on blood-letting and finally a formula for a sudorific, which used sarsaparilla and guaiac wood as the main ingredients.[233] De Baillou also added instructions for an ointment made of the foam of boiling guaiac and sarsaparilla, and besides this, even an ointment made of mercury was recommended. However, mercury also appeared as an ingredient in a formula for pills.[234] Just like to the other consilia, a postscript (Annotatio) of the publisher, the physician Thévart, was added to this consilium. Here he absolutely unequivocally expressed his opinion of mercury: "The panacea for venereal lues is mercury, which is the only thing that defeats this harpy and destroys it ..."[235]

4.5 Summary

The brief outline of the consilia intended for syphilis patients could not be detailed enough and it was not possible to capture and process all aspects and interesting points. A large number of questions that arose in the course of the detailed analysis of the consilia remain as a challenge for further study. Minimal attention was devoted to the great diversity of the typological approach with regards to the three-part structure of the "ideal" consilium. The variety in the structure of individual consilia may in this summary be documented by two of da Monte's consilia for syphilis patients that appear together but have not been mentioned yet. In the first, the longest part is the "casus" with an analysis of maladies, accompanied by plenty of citations from Galen's works with a discussion on the use of baths, while the "cura," meaning the prescription and treatment were resolved with a few words

231 Ballonius, *Consiliorum liber tertius*, 269-70, Cons. CX. Ad luem veneream incipientem.

232 Ibid., 269.

233 Ibid.

234 Ibid., 270.

235 Ibid. "Luis venereae alexiterium est hydrargyrus, hanc hydram solus vincit et opprimit ..." Unnamed opponents however according to what is mentioned only differed on opinions about the nature of the effect of mercury, and didn't protest about its toxicity or use as such.

concerning simple matters and a decoction made of guaiac.[236] The second consilium, where three lines sufficed for the theoretical introduction and prognosis (casus) and the treatment cura included many pages of formulas, schedules of daily dosages and even recommended behavior, is the complete opposite.[237] Issues concerning potential connections and continuity of consilia were also only hinted at, e.g. in Guarinoni's cases, where several consilia likely concerned one patient.[238] It was demonstrated that compared with medical letters, which were not submitted to major editorial changes and in most of which even dates were preserved, uncovering the sequence of events and connections in consilia literature is much more complicated.

However, let us return to the questions that were to be answered as a result of the study of the selected consilia for syphilis patients. Firstly, the number of consilia on the treatment of the French disease on average is surprisingly not at all high. It is however essential to note that but for several exceptions, consilia, where the pox did not figure as the patient's most serious problem, were not taken into account. On the other hand, however, several consilia, where the physicians themselves ruled out the possibility that the patient was suffering from the French disease, were counted. In places, the patient was already cured and in others, he could not even become ill because of his overly cool physical constitution. Illustrative examples are two of da Monte's patients – a Jew, for whom his ethnic origin played a role, and the wife of a syphilis patient, where the results were influenced by her gender, generally considered cooler and moister compared to the temperament of a man.[239] Besides this, the chapter devoted to the origination of collections and anthologies demonstrated that the inclusion of any consilium into a collection depended more or less on chance, the volition of the editor, or the needs of the printer.

The percentage of patients successfully identified thanks to a name, is negligible. In some consilia, it is evident that the name was intentionally withheld, but it does not seem that it occurred more frequently than in cases of other diseases. It is not yet possible to determine how big a role was played by the year of publication here, but the majority of the examined

236 Montanus, *Consultationum opus*, 818-21, Cons. CCCXLIX. De pedum affectione in morbo Gallico, cum pruritu maximo, corpore contabescente, ..., 821. "... nolite ergo ita abhorrere ab his balneis ..."

237 Ibid., 821, Cons. CCCL. De ulceribus cocoethis [sic] gallicis in utroque crure cum tumore splenis, pro iuvene Vicentino.

238 Guarinonius, *Consilia medicinalia*, 32-4, Cons. XXIX.; 39, Cons. XXX.; 44, Cons. XXXI.

239 For more see Montanus, *Consultationum medicarum opus*, 330, Cons. CXXXIII. De catarrho cum suspicione morbi gallici; 861, CCCLXI. De uxore eiusdem laborante ex melancholia et suspicione morbi Gallici.

anthologies were published after the death of the author, so even the syphilis patient concerned could have been dead at the time of publication and physicians did not have to fear negative reactions on the part of the patient or members of his family. In addition to this, professional medical texts written in Latin were only comprehensible and attractive for only a small proportion of the literate public and editors did not have to count on the interest of anyone else but physicians, or scholars from the "Res publica litteraria." The German physician Johann Benedict called upon syphilis patients not to be embarrassed to share intimate symptoms with their physicians, with whom they are safe as with a confessor, (which arouses suspicion that patients were hesitant), but the examined consilia cases do not indicate that physicians threatened the moral stigmatization of their syphilis patients.[240] Perhaps even because of this, physicians like for example Vettori, or the editors of Trincavelli's and da Monte's consilia did not hesitate to designate sexual intercourse as the manner of catching the infection. Da Monte even did so with regards to his own father. This openness could have even sprung from the opinion at the time that regular sexual intercourse represented an essential component in the removal of the bodily humors of a man, the prevention of which would cause harm to him. To what extent sex is essential for men even in the course of the disease was debated immediately after the outbreak of the epidemic and our counsellors, with the exception of da Monte, did rather not to recommend it.[241] However, many physicians did not mention the manner of transmission of the infection in the anamnesis (in many the anamnesis is missing completely) and we mustn't forget that even non-venereal theories via miasma, clothing and dishes were still considered. Recipients of consilia however came from (but for exceptions) the wealthy classes in which certain facts, which could not be passed over unnoticed among less affluent groups, were and are tolerated. Despite this, however, it does not seem that the French disease was looked upon as morally objectionable as strictly as in later centuries.

"The nature of the French disease was always controversial," as physicians themselves admitted, but for the sake of designating the diagnosis and treatment, the author had to at least superficially touch upon these disputed questions and demonstrate his philosophical-medical education and professional perspective.[242] The theory of the occult qualities of the

240 Quetel, *The History of Syphilis*, 26.

241 Arrizabalaga, "Medical Responses," 47-9.

242 He especially interestingly applied himself to the issue of the origination of the pox, their changes and epidemic theory with occult qualities of da Monte, for more see Montanus,

disease, which J. Fernel published in the year 1548, was definitely well known to all of the selected physicians, which is proven by for example comments in da Monte's or Guarinoni's consilia. The ideas about contagions and fomes/fomites from the work of G. Fracastoro also found fertile ground among counsellors, but as was common, their comprehension and connection to other innovations and older theories depended upon the individual decisions of each physician. For example, Venusti in his analysis of the nature of the pox alternately cited both Fernel's and Galen's opinions and it cannot be known whether he inclined more to either one of them.[243] Guarinoni's opinion on the connection between the pox and epilepsy appears completely distinctive.[244] The cause of one disease by the effects of another was not a new medical theory in the early modern period, nevertheless Guarinoni's approach seems to be different.[245] It is however a question whether it is not rather a manifestation of the symptomatological designation of different diseases (scabies = luetic rash, epilepsy = strong cramps), which today causes certain misunderstandings.

A more detailed analysis of the consilia for syphilis patients confirmed the merging of consilia literature with related genres: many of Guarinoni's consilia can be called treatises on the French disease and the same applies to de Baillou; several consilia from da Monte and Trincavelli included interesting "historiae rarae" and observations, and many consilia for syphilis patients can be directly labeled as "epistolae medicinales."[246] It is precisely in these letters, which – put among consilia – did not receive more attention, that many valuable pieces of information both concerning collaboration with colleagues and about patients can be found among the cases of Guarinoni, Solenander, Mermann and Wittich. Thanks to comments in the consilia between Wittich and the consulting Schröter, the fact that they were related was uncovered, which may explain what circumstances

Consultationum medicarum opus, 835-6, CCCLII.; 857-8, Cons. CCCLX.; Capivaccio analyzed the nature of the pox Capivaccius, Opera omnia, 971, Cons. XXVIII. We find an analysis of the differences of temperament between the genders, types of symptoms or manifestations of the French disease in Venustus, *Consilia medica*, 137-43, Cons. IX. Absolutely characteristic and extremely lengthy are the theoretical interpretations of Guarinoni and de Baillou; some of their consilia can even be considered theoretical treatises, meaning non-real consilia. For more see Guarinonius, *Consilia medicinalia*, 393. CCCLXVIII.; Ballonius, *Consiliorum liber secundus*, 185-92.

243 Venustus, *Consilia medica*, 137, Cons. IX.

244 Guarinonius, *Consilia medicinalia*, 17, Cons. XV.; 18, Cons. XVI.; 27, Cons. XXVIII.; 39, XXX.

245 For more on diseases originating from "sympathy," meaning harmony with another disease see Arrizabalaga et al., *The Great Pox*, 236-51; in detail 335, comment no. 55.

246 For "historiae rarae" see e.g. Montanus, *Consultationum opus*, 876, Cons. CCCLXII.; or Trincavellius, *Consilia medica*, 443, Cons. XLIII.

influenced an attending physician in his selection of a counsellor for his patient.[247] The comforting consilium-letter to Solenander's friend captures a close relationship between physician and patient and tells us a lot about the internal feelings of the patient, which we would never learn anything about from a typical professional consilium.[248] This consilium also mentions the evidently common practice of colleagues standing in for one another if another member of the medical staff (court and certainly also faculty) was away from the workplace for professional or personal reasons.[249] One can assume that Solenander occasionally repaid the favor to Weyer.

Collegial collaboration or assistance is the fundamental idea of consilia literature and took place in every consilium contact (if only in writing) between the requestor and counsellor. The final appeals from Venusti's and Mermann's consilia, where both asked the attending physicians to send feedback, attest to the importance of the role that consilia played in connecting members of the Respublica medica.[250] Many notes which could add to our knowledge about the network of contacts between early modern physicians appear right in the text. Da Monte mentioned his own personal collaboration with Girolamo Fracastoro. The consilium in which he acknowledged Fracastoro and his opinion on mercury, was certainly written before the year 1548, when their friendship suffered a serious rift.[251] Valuable are not only mentions of famous figures, but no less important is the name of a physician entirely unknown today mentioned by Vettori, Hieronymus Drogo.[252] The patient of this doctor held a prestigious position, so it is unlikely that he would have chosen an insignificant novice as his personal physician. It may only be a matter of time before historians learn more about H. Drogo, and even the mention from the consilium may play a role in the identification of his name in connection with the correspondence network of the rei publicae medicae. Even the biographical information of A. M. Venusti, who in his consilium for a syphilis patient recommended the works of his teachers Gabriele Falloppio and Antonio Fracanzani, could be

247 Wittichius, *Medicorum consilia*, 550.

248 Solenander, *Consiliorum medicinalium sectiones*, Section V., 493-98, Cons. XVII.

249 For example, at the Imperial Court physicians had the right to paid or if necessary unpaid vacation during which naturally someone had to fill in for them. For more see Hausenblásová, *Der Hof Kaisers Rudolfs II.*, 103.

250 Venustus, *Consilia medica*, 143; Mermannus, *Consultationes*, 501.

251 Girolamo Fracastoro was Montanus's 11-year older countryman, so it would be surprising if they did not know one another. In the year 1548, they got into a dispute because of Montanus's criticism of Fracastoro's work on infectious diseases.

252 Victorius, *Medicinalia consilia*, 1556, 5r., Consilium I.

completed.[253] These professors taught together in Padua, so it will be possible to slightly modify Venusti's scanty biography containing information that he studied in Bologna.[254]

In consilia, we encountered frequent criticism of the previous treatment of the patient. Most often, the greediness of colleagues, which was criticized by for example Capivaccio, de Baillou, or Guarinoni, who also "ex post" denounced the failure to follow his instructions by the attending physician, played a role. If multiple physicians from a faculty council had to agree upon a consilium, it is natural that conflicts sometimes occurred, especially in disputable diagnoses. This manifested itself in several of da Monte's consilia and even more clearly in the collections of Trincavelli and Capivaccio, where the consilia of at least two physicians are captured in multiple cases. Not only did physicians in consilia occasionally disagree on the diagnosis, but they also differed – perhaps only in details – in their approach to treatment. They clearly expected that the practical use of the advice from the consilium would be managed by the patient's attending physician, and even he perhaps lost sleep on account of the advice of colleagues. The majority of the consilia examined prove that the practical application of the conclusions of a consilium, or even several consilia at once, was not an enviable task. Even the conclusions upon which the medical council agreed occasionally remind one of the fabled oracles of Apollo. However, we cannot say whether the possible lack of clarity is due to an inaccurate or incomplete record of a consilium, or editorial changes. It is altogether certain that less-than-clear advice occasionally elicited a response from attending physicians in further requests for clarification, and in this way the correspondence connections between members of the "Respublica litteraria" could continue to develop effectively. Besides disputes and conflicts between colleagues, reservations regarding competing professions also appeared. For example, da Monte criticized a surgeon for overusing mercury in treatment, and the same thing bothered him about the Empiricists, whom he denounced. Capivaccio discontentedly mentioned a Jew who advised treating gonorrhea with sexual intercourse.[255]

Preparations used in the course of treatment were indicated to a limited extent, while the primary topic became the duel between the two main medications for fighting the French disease. In the selected consilia, guaiac

253 Venustus, *Consilia medica*, 142, Cons. IX.

254 Hirsch, *Biographisches Lexikon*, 86-7.

255 For more on these groups of healers see Gentilcore, "Charlatans, the Regulated Marketplace and the Treatment," 57-80; Quetel, *The History of Syphilis*, 86-93.

wood clearly came out on top and was only left out in several individual cases, where the physicians Venusti, Capivaccio, Guarinoni and Crato feared its overly powerful effects, or connected drastic diets. The faith in the strength of guaiac was so great that Vettori and Trincavelli recommended using guaiacum to patients only in the event that the lighter treatment failed, while da Monte and Guarinoni considered it an absolutely essential ingredient.

Of the selected physicians, none used mercury in his consilia as the main means of treatment, and the majority called mercury too dangerous. Of course, even here differences in individual approaches appeared: da Monte literally cursed it and Crato warned against it, while Trincavelli recommended adding mercury vapor to a guaiac decoction and apparently occasionally used a mercury ointment. Both Guarinoni and Solenander also recognized the positive effects of mercury in external use for dermal problems and Wittich used mercury as a component of laxatives. Although de Baillou spoke of mercury as a panacea, he only prescribed it to his patients in the form of a mercury ointment, while Mermann called attention to the successful internal use of "mercurius praecipitatus." An unreservedly positive attitude towards mercury can finally be found in the annotations to de Baillou's consilium, which was written in the year 1643 by de Baillou's editor Thévart, who considered the internal use of mercury to be the only reliable means for treating the pox. It is confirmed that in the 16th century it was not a question of using guaiacum or mercury, but guaiacum and mercury. However, all the selected physicians in their consilia unequivocally preferred guaiacum, thus one cannot fully concur with the assumption that guaiacum was already on the decline starting in the 1560s.[256]

It is possible that the rejection of mercury was influenced by its use by Empiricists and barber-surgeons, who were always – as we have seen in the consilia – accused of its excessive use.[257] Erudite physicians tried to avoid adopting empiric medicaments, and although even guaiacum was one of these and some erudite physicians started to view Empiricists and empiric experience more amiably (recall Guarinoni's positive comments) in the second half of the 16th century, efforts of physicians to separate themselves from other groups of healers clearly continued.[258] Guaiacum thus only lost its privileged status in the course of the first half of the 17th century.

256 Porter, *The Greatest Benefit*, 194.

257 For more see French and Arrizabalaga, "Coping with the French Disease, " 273. Erudite physicians defended themselves.

258 Ibid., 255-7.

Research of the consilia and consultations of the 17th century could provide a more exact determination of when treatment using mercury started to dominate in practice.

As well as mercury and guaiac, several other less common aspects of modern medicine were also mentioned briefly. First, let us make a stop at astrology and the so-called black and white magic.[259] In his consilia, Cristoforo Guarinoni mentioned these influences most frequently and in the greatest detail. In connection with the treatment of great pox, he made – as did Trincavelli – several interesting comments concerning exorcism and further about the use of amulets and incantations, which were supposed to provide relief to the patient and belonged to white magic.[260] For a change, several colleagues of Trincavelli discussed black magic and the use of magic to cause disease, nevertheless this option was rejected by all the participating physicians.[261] Accusations of intentionally causing the French disease by means of incantations and spells figured at the same time in many legal actions resolved by court trials.[262] Another means of treatment included beside common procedures and medication, were spas. They were recommended by Vettori, da Monte and Solenander as well as the renowned Paduan professors Capivaccio and Mercuriale, who in the case of their important patient – according to Guarinoni's testimony – imprudently pushed for him to stay at the spa in Padua. Many expert works were written concerning thermal springs, and spas experienced a significant boom in the 16th century. Drinking cures and baths that were used in the treatment of the French disease corresponded completely with the principles of humoral theory, nevertheless it would be interesting to determine what other spa visitors had to say about the treatment of these patients, since in Paris even lepers protested against the placement of syphilis patients near the leprosarium.[263]

We will now conclude the enumeration of details and information of interest to the historian. It would be possible to continue, however an absolutely detailed analysis was not the objective. On a general level, it would be possible in summary to say that as expected, no shocking thoughts or radical revelations, which would force us to modify and rewrite the current valid definition of consilia literature or the facts concerning the history

259 For more e.g. Robert Jütte, *Krankheit und Gesundheit in der frühen Neuzeit* (Stuttgart: Kohlhammer Verlag, 2013),139-42.

260 Trincavellius, *Consilia medica*, 443, Cons. XLIII.

261 Ibid., 442, 444.

262 For more about cases of (exclusively) women accused of "conjuring up" the French disease see McGough, *Gender*, 88-9.

263 For more see Quetel, *The History of Syphilis*, 24-5.

of the French disease, appeared in the approaches to treatment and ideas which physicians expressed. If the data which historians J. Arrizabalaga or R. French arrived at after studying the earliest medical records concerning this disease, and the conclusions stemming from early modern consilia for syphilis patients, were compared, one could say that they correspond to one another almost 100%. However, as was hinted at in the introduction to this part of the study, in the one hundred years since the outbreak of the lues epidemic, contemporary physicians were unable to escape its shadow and break free of the pattern of medical theory that was to apply up until the beginning of the 19th century.

Bibliography

Arrizabalaga, Jon, John Henderson, and Roger French. *The Great Pox. The French Disease in Renaissance Europe.* New Haven: Yale University Press, 1997.

Arrizabalaga, Jon. "Medical Responses to the 'French Disease' in Europe at the Turn of the Sixteenth Century." In *Sins of the Flesh. Responding to Sexual Disease in Early Modern Europe*, edited by Kevin Siena, 35-55. Toronto: Centre for Reformation and Renaissance Studies, 2005.

Arrizabalaga, Jon. "Problematizing Retrospective Diagnosis in the History of Disease," *Asclepio* 54, no. 1 (2002): 51-70.

Ballonius, Gulielmus. *Consiliorum medicinalium liber primus.* Paris: Iacobus Quesnel, 1635.

Ballonius, Gulielmus. *Consiliorum medicinalium liber secundus.* Paris: Iacobus Quesnel, 1635.

Ballonius, Gulielmus. *Consiliorum medicinalium liber tertius et postremus, item paradigmata et historiae morborum ob raritatem observatione dignissimae.* Paris: Iacobus Quesnel, 1649.

Bloch, Iwan. *Der Ursprung der Syphilis.* Jena: Fischer, 1901.

Brandt, Allan M. "Sexually Transmitted Diseases," In *Companion Encyclopedia of the History of Medicine,* eds. William F. Bynum, and Roy Porter, 562-6. London: Routledge, 1993.

Brown, Kevin. *The Pox. The Life and Near Death of a Very Social Disease.* Thrupp: History Press, 2006.

Bylebyl, Jerom J. "The Manifest and the Hidden in the Renaissance Clinic." In *Medicine and the Five Senses*, edited by William. F. Bynum, and Roy Porter, 40-60. Cambridge: Cambridge University Press, 1993.

Capivaccius, Hieronymus. *Opera omnia ... qua editione, tum Capivaccii plurima typis hactenus novum vulgata in lucem proferuntur.* Frankfurt am Main: Paltheniana, 1603.

Černý, Karel. "Mezi Fracastorem, Fernelem a Helmontem: původ a dynamika vývoje epidemie syfilis v lékařské literatuře 16. a 17. století" [Between Fracastoro, Fernel and Helmont: The Origin and Dynamics of the Development of the Syphilis Epidemic in medical Literature of the 16th and 17th Centuries], *Česká dermatovenerologie* 2, no. 1 (2012): 28-30.

Černý, Karel. "Problém retrospektivní diagnostiky v dějinách lékařství" [The Problem of Retrospective Diagnosis in the History of Medicine], *Dějiny věd a techniky* [*History of Sciences and Technology*] 41, no. 3 (2008): 145-54.

Černý, Karel. *Mor 1480-1730. Epidemie v lékařských traktátech raného novověku* [*The Plague 1480-1730. Epidemics in Early Modern Medical Treatises*]. Prague: Karolinum, 2014.

Crato a Kraftheim, Ioannes. *Consiliorum et epistolarum medicinalium liber quintus.* Frankfurt am Main: Andreae Wecheli heredes, 1594.

Crato a Kraftheim, Ioannes. *Consiliorum et epistolarum medicinalium liber sextus.* Hanau: haeredes Ioannis Aubrii, 1611.

Cunningham, Andrew, and Ole P. Grell. *The Four Horsemen of the Apokalypse. Religion, War, Famine and Death in Reformation Europe.* Cambridge: Cambridge University Press, 2000.

Cunningham, Andrew. "Identifying Diseases in the Past: Cutting through the Gordian Knot," *Asclepio* 54, no. 1 (2002): 13-34.

D'Andrea, David M., *Civic Christianity in Renaissance Italy. The Hospital of Treviso 1400-1530.* Rochester: University of Rochester Press, 2007.

De Renzi, Silvia. "The Great Pox." In *Health, Disease and Society in Europe 1500-1800,* edited by Peter Elmer, and Ole P Grell, *146-50.* Manchester: Manchester University Press, 2004.

Divišová, Bohdana. "Problematika syfilis očima lékaře Christophora Guarinoniho (1534-1604)" [The Problems of Syphilis through the Eyes of Physician Christophoro Guarinoni], *Dějiny věd a techniky* [*History of Sciences and Technology*] 46, no. 2 (2013): 94-112.

Eamon, Wiliam. *"Cannibalism and contagion: framing syphilis in Counter-Reformation Italy," Early Science and Medicine 3, no. 2 (1998): 1-31.*

Eamon, William. *The Professor of Secrets. Mystery, Medicine, and Alchemy in Renaissance Italy.* Washington: National Geographic, 2010.

Eckart, Wolfgang U., and Robert Jütte. *Medizingeschichte. Eine Einführung.* Cologne: Böhlau Verlag, 2007.

Fernelius, Ioannes. *Consiliorum medicinalium liber, cui accesserunt responsa quaedam.* Leiden: Thomas Soubron et Moysen de Prez, 1597.

Fernellius, Ioannes. *Consiliorum liber, cui accesserunt responsa quaedam clarorum medicorum Parisiensium.* Paris: Aegidius Beysius, 1585.

Fernellius, Ioannes. *Consiliorum medicinalium liber. Ex eius adversariis quadringentarum consultationum selectus.* Paris: Aegidius Beysius, 1582.

Fernelius, Ioannes. *Consiliorum medicinalium liber quadringentarum consultationum selectus.* Turin: Gio. Dominicus Tarinus, 1589.

Forrester, John M., and John Henry. *Jean Fernel's On the Hidden Causes of Things: Forms, Souls, and Occult Disease in Renaissance Medicine.* Leiden: Brill, 2005.

Fracastoro, Girolamo. *Syphilis sive morbus gallicus.* Basel: Palma Beb., 1536.

French, Roger, and Jon Arrizabalaga. "Coping with the French Disease: University Practitioners' Strategies and Tactics in the Transition from the Fifteenth to the Sixteenth Century." In *Sins of the Flesh. Responing to Sexual Disease in Early Modern Europe, edited by Kevin Siena,* 248-87. *Toronto:* Centre for Reformation and Renaissance Studies, 2005.

Gallus, Paschalis. *Bibliotheca medica. Sive catalogus illorum, qui ex professo artem medicam in hunc usque annum scriptis illustraruntur.* Basel: Conradus Waldkirch, 1590.

Gentilcore, David. "Charlatans, the Regulated Marketplace and the Treatment of Venereal Disease in Italy." In *Sins of the Flesh. Responding to Sexual Disease in Early Modern Europe,* edited by Kevin Siena, 57-80. Toronto: Centre for Reformation and Renaissance Studies, 2005.

Gentilcore, David. *Medical Charlatanism in Early Modern Italy.* Oxford: Oxford University Press, 2006.

Grafton, Anthony, April Shelford, and Nancy G. Siraisi. *New World, Ancient Texts. The Power of Tradition and the Shock of Discovery.* Cambridge (MA): The Belknap Press, 1992.

Guarinonius, Christophorus. *Consilia medicinalia, in quibus universa praxis medica exacte pertractatur.* Venice: Thoma Baglioni, 1610.

Hausenblásová, Jaroslava. *Der Hof Kaisers Rudolfs II. Eine Edition der Hofstaatsverzeichnisse 1576-1612.* Prague: Artefactum, 2002.

Hayton, Darin. *"Joseph Grünpeck's Astrological Explanation of the French Disease."* In *Sins of the Flesh. Responding to Sexual Disease in Early Modern Europe,* edited by Kevin Siena, *81-108.* Toronto: Centre for Reformation and Renaissance Studies, 2005.

Henderson, John. *The Renaissance Hospital. Healing the Body and Healing the Soul.* New Haven: Yale University Press, 2006.

Hirsch, August, ed. *Biographisches Lexikon der hervorragenden Aerzte aller Zeiten und Völker,* 6., Wien-Leipzig: Urban und Schwarzenberg, 1888.

https://www.treccani.it/enciclopedia/bernardo-cles_%28Dizionario-Biografico%29/ (2.11.2020)

Jütte, Robert. "Syphilis and Confinement: Hospitals in Early Modern Germany." In *Institutions of Confinement: Hospitals, Asylums, and Prisons in Western Europe and North America, 1500-1950*, edited by Norbert Finzsch, and Robert Jütte, 97-115. Cambridge: Cambridge University Press, 1996.

Jütte, Robert. *Krankheit und Gesundheit in der Frühen Neuzeit*. Stuttgart: Kohlhammer Verlag, 2013.

Karenberg, Axel. "Retrospective Diagnosis: Use and Abuse in Medical Historiography," *Prague Medical Report* 110, no. 2 (2009): 140-45.

Kusukawa, Sachiko. "The medical knowledge of the ancient Greeks." In *The Healing Arts: Health, Disease and Society in Europe 1500-1800, edited by Peter Elmer, 5-11. Manchester: Manchester University Press, 2004.*

Lindemann, Mary, *Medicine and Society in Early Modern Europe*, Cambridge: Cambridge University Press, 2010.

Lindenius, Ioannes Antonides. *De scriptis medicis libri duo*. Amsterdam: Iohannes Blaev, 1637.

McGough, Laura J. *Gender, Sexuality, and Syphilis in Early Modern Venice: the Disease that Came to Stay*. Basingstoke: Palgrave Macmillan, 2010.

Mermannus, Thomas. *Consultationes ac responsiones medicae*. Ingolstadt: Joannes Phillippus Zinck, 1675.

Montanus, Ioannes Baptista. *Consultationum medicarum opus absolutissimum*. Basel: Petri, 1565.

Nicolson, Malcolm. "The Art of Diagnosis: Medicine and the Five Senses." In *Companion Encyclopedia of the History of Medicine,* edited by William F. Bynum, and Roy Porter, 801-18. London: Routledge, 1993.

Nutton, Vivian. "Humoralism." In *Companion Encyclopedia of the History of Medicine,* eds. William F. Bynum, and Roy Porter, 281-91. London: Routledge, 1993.

Nutton, Vivian. "The Reception of Fracastoro's Theory of Contagion: The Seeds That Fell among Thorns?," *Osiris* 6 (1990): 196-243.

Ongaro, Giuseppe, and Elda Martellozzo Forin. "Girolamo Mercuriale e lo studio di Padova." In *Girolamo Mercuriale. Medicina e cultura nell'Europa del cinquecento,* edited by Alessandro Arcangeli, and Vivian Nutton, 29-50. Firenze: L.S. Olschki, 2008.

Ortner, Donald J. *Identification of Pathological Conditions in Human Skeletal Remains*. Amsterdam: Academic Press, 2003.

Pelling, Margaret. "Contagion/Germ Theory/Specificity." In *Companion Encyclopedia of the History of Medicine,* edited by William F. Bynum, and Roy Porter, 309-19. London: Routledge, 1993.

Porter, Roy. *The Greatest Benefit to Mankind. A Medical History of Humanity from Antiquity to the Present.* London: Harper Collins Publishers, 1997.

Priesner, Claus, and Karin Figala, eds. *Alchemie. Lexikon einer hermetischen Wissenschaft*. Munich: Verlag C.H.Beck Ohg., 1998.

Quetel, Claude. *The History of Syphilis*. Baltimore: John Hopkins University Press, 1990.

Rill, Gerhard di. “Cles, Bernardo,” *Dizionario Biografico degli Italiani*, 26 (1982).

Rütten, Thomas. “Early Modern Medicine.” In *The Oxford Handbook of the History of Medicine*, edited by Mark Jackson, 60-81. Oxford: Oxford University Press, 2011.

Schenckius, Ioannes Georgius. *Biblia iatrica sive bibliotheca medica macta, continuata.* Frankfurt am Mein: Ioannes Spiess, 1609.

Schleiner, Winfried. “Infection and Cure through Women: Renaissance Constructions of Syphilis,” *Journal of Medieval and Renaisance Studies* 24, no. 3 (1994): 499-17.

Scholzius, Laurentius. *Consiliorum medicinalium, conscriptorum a praestantissimis atque exercitatissimis nostrorum temporum medicis liber singularis.* Frankfurt am Mein: Andreae Wecheli Haeredes, 1598.

Sherrington, Charles. *The Endeavour of Jean Fernel*, Cambridge: Cambridge University Press, 1946.

Siraisi, Nancy G. “Giovanni Argenterio: Medical innovation, princely patronage, and academic controversy.” In *Medicine and the Italian Universities 1250-1600*, edited by Nancy G. Siraisi, 328-55. Leiden: Brill 2001.

Solenander, Reinerus. *Consiliorum medicinalium sectiones quinque.* Frankfurt am Mein: Andreae Wecheli heredes, 1596.

Stein, Claudia. *Die Behandlung der Franzosenkrankheit in der Frühen Neuzeit am Beispiel Augsburg.* Stuttgart: Franz Steiner Verlag, 2003.

Stein, Claudia. *Negotiating the French Pox in Early Modern Germany.* Farnham: Ashgate Press, 2009.

Stolberg, Michael. *Die Harnschau. Eine Kultur-und Alltagsgeschichte.* Cologne: Böhlau Verlag, 2009.

Stolberg, Michael. *Homo patiens. Krankheits-und Körpererfahrung in der frühen Neuzeit.* Cologne: Böhlau Verlag, 2003.

Torella, Gaspare. *Tractatus cum consiliis contra pudendagram.* Romae: Petrus de la Turre, 1497.

Trincavellius, Victor. *Consilia medica post editionem Venetam et Lugdunensem.* Basel: Conradus Valdkirchius, 1587.

Trincavellius, Victor. *Consiliorum medicinalium libri tres; Epistolarum medicinalium libri tres.* Venice: Camillus Borgominerius, 1586.

Venustus, Antonius Maria. *Consilia medica.* Venice: Franciscus Zilettus, 1571.

Victorius, Benedictus. *Consilia medicinalia, ad varia morborum genera.* Venice: Iordan Zillettus, 1556.

Webster, Charles. *Paracelsus: Medicine, Magic and Mission at the End of Time.* New Haven: Yale University Press, 2008.

Wittichius, Iohannes. *Nobilissimorum ac Doctissimorum Germaniae Medicorum consilia, observationes atque epistolae medicae.* Leipzig: Henning Grossius, 1604.

5 Conclusion

Abstract

The study is based primarily on the works of fifteen physicians under whose names 22 collections or anthologies of consilia were published. The representatives of Italian, German and French medicine held various positions in the professional hierarchy (professors, personal physicians, municipal physicians). After a general introduction to the approaches to their publications and the contents of these collections and anthologies, consilia that focused on the treatment of the great pox were selected in order to uncover potential details and specific features. It has been demonstrated that consilia, like observation or medical correspondence, represented an important link between the members of the forming Respublica medica.

Keywords: consilia, physicians, patients, collaboration, Respublica medica

> "Seeking medical advice by letter from high-profile physicians was by no means an unknown practice in early modern Europe. ... However, the practice in France has been somewhat neglected by medical historians."[1]

Although R. Weston meant a period somewhat later with these words, his comments also fully apply to consilia of the 16th century, and not only for France. Consilia did not escape the attention of historians engaged in the epistemology of the early modern period at all, but they do not figure as the main topic. They rather constitute a supplementary background in the study and definition of the boundaries of related genres. Awareness of consilia literature of the 16th century as a genre itself remains superficial and we lack especially constituent works covering exclusively the consilia of specific regions, publishers, or individual authors.

The present study was intended as far as possible as a continuation of the work on medieval consilia literature and to supplement current studies

1 Weston, *Medical Consulting*, 1.

Divišová, Bohdana, *Medical Case Studies (Consilia medica) of the Early Modern Period.*
Taylor & Francis Group, 2022
doi: 10.5117/9789463723640_ch05

concerning related case history genres. 22 collections and anthologies of consilia of 16th-century physicians that were published in print constituted the foundation. The result however is not completely exhaustive, and many particular topics were not even mentioned, while some were just hinted at. These include, for example, the detailed differences in the form and content of the various types of consilia that we came across – classic consilia sent in the form of a letter by a single physician, consilia of members of a faculty of medicine, or consilia that were student records of clinical instruction at a hospital or private home. Especially the last-mentioned type of consilia deserves closer attention. The presence of students and instruction certainly had an influence on the behavior of the consulting professors, the course of the medical consultation and even the form of the resulting record. Research into these details will require more time and both a broader and more in-depth scope of study. It is however likely that archival materials will be found more helpful for answering the majority of questions. Due to editorial revisions before printing, it is often not possible to even determine whether the consultation letter, supplemental record of the consultation, or the description of instruction of students was edited.

However, consilia published in print represent only a fraction of the total produced. Unfortunately, we cannot estimate how great a fraction this is. Many consilia were likely not preserved because not every consulting physician or patient saved the delivered consilium, and many consilia certainly remain hidden in the manuscript departments of various European archives. A more careful study of all related genres of medical literature will very likely show that many consilia are hidden or were published under the name of a related genre. As we have noted, all early modern medical genres devoted to case studies overlap one another, so in the study of one, it is not possible to omit the others.

An absolute majority of the collections or anthologies of consilia of the chosen authors were published at a time that I. Maclean described as a period characterized by the maximum flowering of the Frankfurt book fairs, common availability of Latin translations of the works of Galen and Hippocrates, and above all the consolidation of the professional medical book market.[2] All of these factors also influenced the development and spread of consilia literature. There can be no doubt that collections and anthologies of consilia successfully joined the other early modern medical genres and successfully competed with them and merged with them.

2 Maclean, *Learning and the Market Place*, 61-2.

Professional medical literature fulfilled an important function which G. Pomata aptly characterized. "As shared textual conventions, genres are intrinsically social: contributing to a genre means consciously joining a community ... some genres are eminently instruments of community building tools for the establishment of a collective scholarly endeavor as a social and intellectual shared space."[3] It is evident that the number of physicians who sought to join in the communication within their elite community continued to grow. Which, that in the middle of the 17th century I. F. Thiermair called a pathological compulsion, was just a strengthening expression of interest in active membership in the Respublica medica. Among physicians from the lower levels of the hierarchy, it could also have been an effort to improve their reputations by means of print.[4] Gaining the awareness of the academic community with an expert treatise was certainly more difficult than contributing to an anthology or periodical with an interesting case from practice, consilium or letter of a renowned colleague.[5]

The initial purpose of a consilium was however to help cure a patient. For understandable reasons, physicians put in print cases of patients whose names added luster to their careers. As has been documented however, the publication of consilia could not have been purely about self-promotion and business on the part of physicians. What benefit was however provided by a consilium in which the result was not recorded, and the reader could thus not verify the efficacy of the recommended formulas? Many consilia even noted the death of the patient which tends to be evaluated as a failure of the physician. In such cases, was not the consilium rather negative publicity? It is difficult to answer such questions. First of all, it was usual for a physician to insure himself in case of failure with a prognosis that in complicated cases was from very cautious to unfavorable. In addition to this, it was impossible to verify (at the very least in cases of actual "remote advice") whether instructions from consilia were followed exactly. In consilia, one can relatively often come across counsellors' reproaches of irresponsible colleagues and disobedient patients. It was also never certain that the pharmacist followed the instructions, used ingredients of suitable quality,

3 Pomata, *Observation Rising*, 48.

4 P. Savoia noticed in his work on surgery at the University of Bologna that of the professors only those from the lower classes published zealously, while the professors originating from elite families did not need to be visible in this way. Savoia, "Skills, Knowledge, and Status," 41-2.

5 At times, of course, the counsellor's response was not positive. J. Crato rejected the request of his friend Thomas Jordan in the letter in an unpleasant way: "De aegro tuo quid scribam? Satis mihi hic est molestiarum." Crato, *Consiliorum liber quartus*, 400.

used the correct ingredients, the medicine was stored properly, and so on. Last but not least, unexpected supernatural events or astrological influences could have been at fault. For a tolerant attitude towards consilia that ended tragically, an important prerequisite was that the treatment approach which failed in one case could work on another patient. The physician could have just been inspired by the approach described and "tailored" the prescription and regimen for a patient with a similar temperament and problems, so that the result was satisfactory. This also helped to drive the unrelenting popularity of consilia.

Collections of consilia were important proof of success for their authors and increased their prestige. To obtain the widest readership among European scholars and ensure the greatest demand, both collections and anthologies of consilia were usually published in Latin. Consilia written in vernacular languages were generally translated for print publication. The preferential use of Latin was also influenced by the status of the patient, who stood somewhat aside in the course of communication between physicians. This situation gradually changed, as indicated by manuscript consultations of the 17th and 18th centuries in which one can discern a growing struggle of the patient for self-determination, enabled by the improving education of classes not belonging to the elite of society.[6]

The creation and printing of consilia were instigated by the growing interest of physicians in case history studies. The importance that physicians at the time attached to following current medical practice ensured the long-term popularity of consilia and consultations. A closer connection with personal experience caused a certain dissatisfaction of physicians with the diagnosing of diseases without personal examination of the patient. Concerns about the correctness of diagnosis without examination were expressed by, for example, V. Trincavelli, a generation younger T. Mermann or C. Guarinoni.[7] Although these physicians are in the minority with their reservations regarding consultations "from afar," at least among the selected representatives of the 16th century, they certainly were not the only ones. L. Scholz's fiery defense of consilia literature testifies to the widespread criticism of therapy "in absentia."[8] Note that evidently even some patients began to evince this trend, as we know thanks to one of the

6 Wild, *Medicine-by-Post*, 9; Kinzelbach et al., "Observationes et Curationes Nurimbergenses," 180; Pilloud, "Interpretationsspielräume und narrative Autorität," 60.

7 Trincavellius, *Consiliorum libri*, 61v., Cons. LII.; Mermannus, *Consultationes*, 243, Cons. IV.; 500, Cons. XVI. pg. 500; Guarinonius, *Consilia medicinalia*, 105, Cons. XCII.

8 Scholzius, *Consiliorum liber singularis*, 3v.

few published request letters, where a patient of R. Solenander refused a written consilium.[9] It however does not seem that the numbers of consilia and consultations sharply declined due to these opinions. Although at the beginning of the 18th century professor of medicine Antonio Vallisneri lamented that "difficile est curare per literas" he very actively cultivated consilia literature.[10]

Let us now return from the 18th century back to the main topic of the study, the works of fifteen physicians under whose names collections or anthologies of consilia were published. Note that the selection of historical figures was not limited to representatives of one school or nationality, but the common link became the fact that during their lifetimes, they achieved such a degree of success that they were asked for advice by their contemporaries. These representatives of Italian, German and French medicine stood at various positions in the professional hierarchy. An absolute majority of them started their careers as municipal physicians or private general practitioners. However, only two of the selected physicians remained true to this role, while the rest climbed higher on the proverbial ladder: seven as professors taught medicine at one of the important faculties of medicine and several of them were then promoted to (even better paid) positions as personal physicians of members of European ruling families. Six of the selected physicians worked their entire lives in this capacity, nevertheless, nothing prevented the accumulation of posts so three managed to hold the posts of both professor and personal physician.

After overall familiarization with the approaches to the publications and contents of the collections of this group of physicians, the study turned to consilia that focused on the treatment of one specific disease called "morbus gallicus." Since the French disease was not to become the main topic of the study, but was to serve only to demonstrate the most interesting moments matching those on which I generally focused in my treatment of the collections and anthologies of consilia, only the most basic facts from the history of this disease were mentioned. In the schematic depiction of the history of this disease, there of course was not more space for many details regarding the specific reactions of physicians, individual communities, or countries. The question of the view of the culprits and a different approach towards their victims, changes in the treatment of syphilis patients brought on by the Reformation, or the influence of the Counter-Reformation campaign of the Catholic Church and other details have been left out. Tracing of the

9 Solenander, *Consiliorum medicinalium sectiones,* 235, Cons. VIII.

10 Gemelli, "Die Sprache der Krankheit," 68.

development of the disease and its treatment in the subsequent centuries was also not within the scope of the narrowly focused topic of this work. However, anyone wanting to learn more about the development of syphilology and the great discoveries of the 19th and 20th centuries, the name August von Wassermann with a description of his serodiagnostic method, Paul Ehrlich and his salvarsan, or Alexander Fleming and the discovery of antibiotics can find this information in every general guide to the history of medicine, specialized treatises and of course on the internet.

A closer look confirmed that rather static discourse, which in many ways is no different from the medieval, is a characteristic of early modern consilia, and the influence of early modern medical-philosophical trends in consilia for syphilis patients cannot be overlooked. Of the innovators of the Galenic-Hippocratic system, among the authors of consilia, Jean Fernel and his teachings concerning occult qualities were most strongly asserted. Although the ideas of Girolamo Fracastoro concerning the seeds of contagion and "fomes" proved to be popular and accepted, Fernel's influence was incomparable. It was further confirmed that guaiac wood and mercury shared the top spot in the treatment of the pox, but that physicians preferred guaiacum for the treatment of wealthy patients throughout the 16th century. The selected sample of consilia showed that in the 16th century syphilis did not yet have the negative tinge of sinfulness as in the following centuries, so there was not a sense that concealing the treatment and identity of the patient was so essential. It seems that in the given consilia, the names of syphilis patients appear in essentially the same frequency as in the cases of other diseases.[11] The attempt or need to maintain medical confidentiality grew, as also documented by a comment from J. Schröter to not commit everything about treatment to paper, but was not by any means yet common.[12] This is also confirmed by some consilia where the full name of the patient is mentioned or where the detailed titles enabled the certain identification of the person.

In the concise overview above, some of the findings regarding important figures of 16th century consilia literature and their works have been recapitulated. In this work, I have first and foremost tried to show the possibility of researching the development of medical epistemology of the given period.

11 Although cases in which disputes between physician and patient occurred due to a failure to maintain anonymity are recorded, they concern other diseases such as impotence. Gellner, *Životopis lékaře Borbonia*, 174. In later periods, requirements for maintaining medical secrecy are more frequent.

12 Wittichius, *Medicorum consilia*, 550.

Using analyses of consilia, I have attempted to remind the reader that consilia are found along the boundaries of science, professional practice and education, and after in-depth study, this interconnectedness promises to deliver interesting information. Once more, it must be reiterated that this study could not cover all aspects of early modern consilia literature. Not only has minimal attention been devoted to the consilia of the 17th and 18th centuries, but the information potential of more detail-focused consilia of the 16th century is also yet to be completely exhausted. In conclusion, one may with a certain view from above sum it up with the fact that consilia literature essentially never lost its popularity in any of the following centuries, while only the means and speed of the entire process changed somewhat. Few people in today's world have not experienced a similar situation to that of the humanist A. Dudith, where one would say into a phone: "Advise me quickly doctor!"[13] The participants and form of the act have changed, but the job of the physician – to quicky aid a patient in need – remains the same, so in a way, remote consultations are eternal.

Bibliography

Crato a Kraftheim, Ioannes. *Consiliorum et epistolarum medicinalium liber quartus.* Frankfurt am Main: Andreae Wecheli heredes, 1593.

Crato a Kraftheim, Ioannes. *Consiliorum et epistolarum medicinalium liber tertius.* Frankfurt am Main: Andreae Wecheli heredes, 1592.

Fortis, Raymundus Ioannes. *Consultationum et responsionum medicinalium centuriae quatuor. Accesserunt eiusdem consilia ...* Genova: Sumptibus Leonardi Chovët 1677.

Gellner, Gustav. *Životopis lékaře Borbonia a výklad jeho deníků* [*The Biography of Physican Borbonius and Explanation of his Diaries*]. Prague: Česká akademie věd a umění, 1938.

Gemelli, Benedino. "Die Sprache der Krankheit in der Korrespondenz von Antonio Vallisneri." In *Krankheit in Briefen im deutschen und französischen Sprachraum 17.-21. Jahrhundert*, edited by Martin Dinges, and Vincent Barras, 67-77. Stuttgart: Franz Steiner Verlag, 2007.

Guarinonius, Christophorus. *Consilia medicinalia.* Venice: Thoma Baglioni, 1610.

Kinzelbach, Annemarie, Susanne Grosser, Kay P. Jankrift, and Marion Ruisinger. "Observationes et Curationes Nurimbergenses. The Medical Practice of Johann Christoph Götz (1688-1733)." In *Medical Practice, 1600-1900. Physicians and Their*

13 Crato, *Consiliorum liber tertius*, 262. "Consule in medium mi D[omine] Doctor!"

Patients, edited by Martin Dinges, Kay Peter Jankrift, Sabine Schlegemilch, and Michael Stolberg, 169-87. Leiden: Brill-Rodopi, 2016.

Maclean, Ian. *Learning and the Market Place. Essays in the History of the Early Modern Book.* Leiden: Brill, 2009.

Mermannus, Thomas. *Consultationes ac responsiones medicae.* Ingolstadt: Joannes Phillippus Zinck, 1675.

Pilloud, Séverine. "Interpretationsspielräume und narrative Autorität im autobiographischen Krankheitsbericht." In *Krankheit in Briefen im deutschen und französischen Sprachraum 17.-21.* Jahrhundert, edited by Martin Dinges, and Vincent Barras, 45-65. Stuttgart: Franz Steiner Verlag, 2007.

Pomata, Gianna. "Observation Rising: Birth of an Epistemic Genre, 1500-1650." In *Histories of Scientific Observation,* edited by Lorraine Daston, and Elisabeth Lunbeck, 45-80. Chicago: The University Chicago Press, 2011.

Savoia, Paolo. "Skills, Knowledge, and Status: The Career of an Early Modern Italian Surgeon," *Bulletin of the History of Medicine* 93, no. 1 (2019): 27-54.

Scholzius, Laurentius. *Consiliorum medicinalium, conscriptorum a praestantissimis atque exercitatissimis nostrorum temporum medicis liber singularis.* Frankfurt am Mein: Andreae Wecheli Haeredes, 1598.

Solenander, Reinerus. *Consiliorum medicinalium sectiones quinque.* Frankfurt am Mein: Andreae Wecheli heredes, 1596.

Trincavellius, Victor. *Consiliorum medicinalium libri tres; Epistolarum medicinalium libri tres.* Venice: Camillus Borgominerius, 1586.

Weston, Robert. *Medical Consulting by Letter in France, 1665-1789.* Farnham: Ashgate Press, 2013.

Wild, Wayne. *Medicine-by-Post: the Changing Voice of Illness in Eighteenth-Century British Consultation Letters and Literature.* Amsterdam: Rodopi, 2006.

Wittichius, Iohannes. *Nobilissimorum ... Germaniae Medicorum consilia, observationes atque epistolae medicae.* Leipzig: Henning Grossius, 1604.

6 An Example Case Study from the 16th Century

Consilium CXV. "A Dermal Rash with the French Disease"[1]
Victor Trincavellius. *Consilia medica post editionem Venetam et Lugdunensem, accessione CXXVIII consiliorum locupleta et per locos communes digesta.* Basel: Conradus Valdkirchius (1587): 678-82.

Abstract
The last part of this work consists of the Consilium CXV., "A dermal rash with the French disease," published in the collection *Consilia medica* of the Italian physician Vittore Trincavelli. The translation was supplemented by a brief commentary and explanations where required by the text. More detailed information on some of the medicines used has also been added. The consilium does not contain the three parts of an "ideal" consilium. It is an example of a consilium that has undergone various adjustments due to the edition, e.g. the end of the consilium was cut off in an almost violent way and so on. The task of the translation is to document the common early modern consilium.

Keywords: Trincavelli, therapy, medicals, French disease

Before we advise the noble and distinguished gentleman, it is essential to lay down the sort of foundations upon which the entire rational decomposition of our speech, which we will conduct concerning the problems that

1 The consilium is translated in its entirety despite the fact that the author discusses certain aspects repeatedly. Considerable lengthiness and verbosity appear in particular in the consilia of Italian authors. At the same time, we should note that humanist literature did not yet know the "terminus technicus," and a uniform terminology did not exist. Anatomical, nosological and even botanical terminologies were marked by disorganization and lack of logic, which caused difficulty not only in the translation of information, but especially in its interpretation. In order to aid comprehension, it was necessary to divide very long sentences, in which humanist Latin excels, into shorter sentences and to add certain words for better understanding. These words are in square brackets.

Divišová, Bohdana, *Medical Case Studies (Consilia medica) of the Early Modern Period.*
Taylor & Francis Group, 2022
doi: 10.5117/9789463723640_ch06

afflict him, is based. With regards to the overall constitution of the body, it is of a warm and dry temperature or nature. Even the darker color of the body indicates a certain burned and roasted state of the blood, which is testified to by the gauntness and fragility of the part and readiness, agility and quickness in all actions. All of the other parts do not fully agree with this overall mixture.[2] Firstly – in order to start from the top – the brain is healthily heated, more moist than dry, which is proven by the amounts of excrements that drip down to the lower located parts, primarily the chest and back.[3] These [excrements] are responsible for the catarrh and pain, which is also documented by the predisposition to longer sleep. The liver is strongly heated and also particularly dry to such a degree that it was able to alter the constitution of the entire body to its likeness. This is shown by the amount of burnt fluid [humor] and the veins, which on [this] type of body are voluminous and full of darker blood. This [burnt fluid] overburdens practically the entire body and almost continuously causes a bothersome and permanent rash. I would not consider the heart itself as strongly heated or overly dry. Although the [patient] is probably quick-tempered, as I have been able to judge from both appearance and speech, it nevertheless does not seem to me that he would be a furious person.[4] He is rather of more genial and kind manners and calms down easily. However, his stomach is assuredly cold and moist. This is proven by the slow and rather difficult boiling and frequent phlegm, which exits the mouth together with sputum.[5] However, all of these things are related to the innate constitution of the body, but due to various lifestyle errors, in the previous period, the imbalances of the entire body, liver and stomach have [yet even] increased. The work and tasks to which, as it seems to me, he is very devoted, however dry the body even more, especially its parts that are warm and dry by nature. To this, we may add the frequent, multiple-timed use of various medicaments, mainly however, the relaxing ones and others that dry a lot. [An example] is the decoction of a wood called guaiac with a mixture of numerous medicines, which although cleansing the body, excessively dry, upset and cause the imbalance mainly of the stomach and liver. It [the liver] then

2 "Parts" (partes) were a component of humoral physiology, just like the "actions" (actiones) in the previous sentence.

3 "Excrements" is the designation for the remnants of the four types of bodily digestion, or boiling (see note no. 5)

4 The temperature of individual organs among other things also influenced the nature (in contemporary terminology, temperament) of a person.

5 "Boiling or cooking" (coctio) occurred in the stomach, liver, heart and brain; a different type of excrement came from each.

becomes drier and evidently burnt even the blood and other fluids. [The stomach] in turn is deprived of powers and natural heat, cooled and began to boil worse.[6] One cannot however at all disregard the no-less important fact that [the patient] suffers greatly from the pernicious French disease, which could not be destroyed by any power or great [pg. 679] suffering that the noble gentleman underwent. Once this malignant poison of the pox is imprinted on the liver in the body of the gentleman's nature, that is, of excessive heat and dryness, it [the liver] retains it so firmly that it cannot be removed from there but with enormous effort. This happened to him as he himself admitted. After all, he used a decoction of guaiacum wood, [underwent] numerous and frequent purgation and had ointments applied by which this infection is usually destroyed. He even ingested a decoction of sarsaparilla and adhered to the procedure that must be followed when using these medicines, and after he underwent bloodletting, he was again very carefully purged. Despite this, he was never able to rid himself completely of this plague. Some remnants of that disease and some sort of seeds, which again multiplied and in the end infected the entire body, always remained. In this manner, we have thus described and defined that from which the important and some sort of conclusions, which may best serve our purposes, must be selected. The first will be that the noble gentleman suffers from dripping since cool and phlegmatic matter drips from the head primarily to the muscles of the chest. [It reaches] especially the left part and there expands and causes pain. Secondly, he so often suffers from a rash that he has never been able to rid himself completely of it. Thirdly, he has a rawer, cooler and moister stomach, and thus digests food slowly and with difficulty. This causes the accumulation of large amounts of raw phlegm in the stomach as well as the head. Fourthly, the body is delicate in nature and of a thin texture, thus easily relaxes. It is evident upon what we must lay the foundation for all future discourse. Especially lately, [the patient] was afflicted by two problems: the dripping to his chest and an irritating, exceedingly itchy rash. Currently, the much greater complaints are regarding the rash so we will discuss it first. Its primary cause is a warm and dry imbalance of the liver. This enables the generation of numerous burnt matter, when part of the more delicate and warmer blood is changed into burnt bile with which a lot of delicate, savory and serous phlegm mixes. In order for the nature [of the body] through its natural system to remove these harmful excrements from the blood, it must continuously push this mixture to the surface of

6 Powers (vires) and innate heat (calor nativus, calidum innatum) were components of humoral physiology.

the skin, where after forming those scaly blisters, causes very annoying itching. Even the skin itself probably allows the rash to do this. It itself is transformed by this long-standing and almost constant problem and the matter, which flows upon it for a very long time, and has adopted an imbalance similar to that of the fluid [excrement of the burnt blood]. This [imbalance] spoils and changes even good nourishment into similarly bad fluids. That is another thing that is added to the previous one and is the reason why the issue becomes more complicated. If this is so, then we must determine and designate a treatment and its first goal is a change in that imbalance of the liver. [Furthermore], it is necessary to destroy that French evil in any way possible. That imbalance incessantly continues and the lues is also made stronger by the presence of those unfavorable fluids, so it will be necessary to first purge the body but with simple and gentle medicaments. [pg. 680] In addition to weakening the powers of the stomach, strong and pungent [medicines] also dry out and warm the body. Even if they cleanse, protect and seemingly benefit [the body], they do much more harm since they dissolve the power of innate heat. Gentle and calming pharmaceuticals have proven themselves to me. However, since the substance, which we want to take away, is easier to remove when it is properly prepared and boiled, it is first essential to designate and follow the right manner of eating, so that [the patient] consumes the right foods from which proper blood is created, since if the right kind is being made, blood can repair almost every deficiency in the body. In this case, the diet will be useful: the best of tender meat of for example chickens and young capons, fattened kids, young calves and fresh eggs. If he ever eats fish, they should be those considered the best – among others perch or pike caught in flowing, good waters, and others of this kind, cooked in soup, as they say, or roasted on a grill. Frying in oil is to be avoided. Consumption of savory things is more adverse than beneficial. The copious consumption of spicy things such as onions, leeks, garlic and others of this kind and everything aromatic, which can strongly heat up and dry out, is also harmful. But not even sweets are very useful because as all things baked, they easily change into burnt bile. It is essential to avoid stronger wines completely, which warm one up and easily go to the head and fill it. Because of a cold and raw [= poor boiling] stomach, [the patient] must cut out spicy and young wines. May he drink those that are ripe, but not too strong, rather light, not heavy, not too dark, but lighter or medium in color. Excessive exertion, which warms the body, is adverse for it [the stomach], and also even rapid movement of the head, especially anger and sadness may do a lot of harm. Most beneficial of all is when digestion remains unobstructed either spontaneously, or by means of an expert procedure using enemas. Sleep is adequate as [is shown by] the head and frequent excrement that forms daily. While following such a regimen, it is furthermore necessary to ensure that the body is suitably cleansed. This is most gently achieved if the bowels are first released using calming medications and remove the general excrements, which accumulate and are retained in the stomach, intestines and first veins [leading] from the stomach. For this purpose, I would select one ounce of cassia flowers.[7] If [the patient] did not tolerate it well, I would add a drachma of hiera simplex powder,[8] or half an ounce of ground hyssop, or the same dose of powdered rhubarb, or anise or fennel. If [the patient] could not stand cassia at all, I would use a laxative potion. [For the preparation of] one and a half ounces, I would take in the same amounts at least two ounces of selected mana and relaxing rose syrup, which I would dissolve in an ordinary decoction of fruit.[9] I would then move on to the processing of other kinds of matter that are in veins and the more distant parts. Those expelled from the veins support and worsen the rash. I would achieve this by means of similar syrups as we obtain from simple chicory syrup, from half an ounce of simple fumitories (fumiterra) and [half an ounce] of hops, four ounces of a decoction of borage, endive, wood sorrel or sorrel and may he take these about seven times. Then I would want him to be cleansed using a medicine of the following composition: Take half an ounce of selected senna leaves, simple small branches, 3 drachmas of raisins, two drachmas of the peeled root of a licorice, a small amount of barley grains without hulls, one drachma each of the individual flowers of borages [pg. 681] anchusas, violets and fumitories. Mix and [from this mixture] prepare a decoction in waters from hops, fumitories and chicory, then strain.[10] Take four ounces of this decoction and to it add four scruples rhubarb, half a scruple of squinanth,[11] may they be sprayed with

7 Flos cassiae was the name used by pharmacists of the time; it is the inside of pods of cassia, not the flower.

8 Hiera simplex – a mixture that was usually composed of nine herbal ingredients and had purgative effects.

9 In Europe, weights and measures were not uniform, nevertheless a pound weighed approximately 360g, an ounce approx. 30g, a drachma 4g and a scruple around 1g.
Mana was the sweet-tasting, hardened plant juice of the manna (flowering) ash tree. Cuts into the tree's bark were made at the end of summer and it was necessary to remove impurities from the dried juice.

10 The text of the Latin master copy is not entirely clear, and it seems that it was damaged in the course of copying or printing. For example, it is missing certain information about the amount of added water, etc.

11 Squinanth is an aromatic grass (Herba schoenanthi or Fenum camelorum) imported from East Asia and North Africa. In the past, it was used as a stomachicum.

aromatic wine beforehand and [then] submerge [them] overnight in the above-described decoction. May they be strained in time and may [the rest] be squeezed out. In this may one ounce of selected mana, three ounces of laxative rose syrup and one drachma of "confectio hamech" preparation be dissolved.[12] Mix so a drink may be created. This must be taken early in the morning in the course of five hours before breakfast. The next morning may he take one ounce of rose sugar and the following day as well so that he may get rest from all medicines. It has proven effective to me on the third day when [the patient] indulges in a bath in regular fresh water and immersed in it takes a proper bath. However, I do not want him to excessively warm himself up or for him to sweat too much in it. Then it seems necessary to me to evaluate, whether there are full and dark veins in the body. Since I would then be glad if bloodletting was performed [on him] from the basilic vein, but not too much, six or seven ounces at most. If the veins were not full, I would look to see, whether the hemorrhoidal veins are full in the [appropriate] place. It has proven very effective to me to open those places, which nature selected, and to allow six to seven ounces of blood to flow out. If not even those [veins] are swollen, I would affix smaller cups, which are used by so-called barbers, at least to the back, hips and places with a more pronounced presence of the rash. After the incision, I would remove the amount of blood that I designated previously so that the defective blood, which causes the dermal problems, flows out. I would not be satisfied with the previous purgation and would again prepare [the patient] for another purgation using these syrups: Take syrups composed of one ounce of fumitories, half an ounce of chicory prepared without rhubarb, four ounces of a decoction made of hops, fumitories and borage and mix. May he use these until the fifth day. Then, may the same medicine, which I described a while ago, be repeated, and the following day after consumption of sugar and the rest like before, may he rest. Then, I would prepare another bath, not a simple one like the first, but I would use mallow, fumitories, borage, sorrel, liverworts, which are called "hepatics," barley without the hull, bran,[13] roots

12 "Confectiones" were solid preparations covered in sugar. "Confectio Hamech" were first mentioned by the Persian physician Mesue (+857). It was a medicine composed of a large number of plant drugs and whey; in each period, the formula was comprised of a different number of ingredients, usually between twenty and forty. Its preparation was extremely complicated and demanding, just as complicated as the preparation of theriac. The attending physician had to decide which composition of the medicine to select.

13 The Latin term "furfur" could among other things have meant flour. The attending physician had to decide what his colleague had in mind and also add missing information concerning the parent plant.

of black hellebore, a handful of each. Firstly, may the barley be cooked until the grains crack, then may the black hellebore and finally the herbs be added. May a bath be prepared from the cooked mixture and may he wash his entire body not once, but repeatedly. However, if after all of this it will seem that he [the patient] has not recovered, – it seems that neither a decoction of guaiacum wood, nor a decoction of sarsaparilla did succeed before, – I would be of the opinion that something of this should be repeated. Many times have I seen that someone could not be cured by the repeated drinking of one of these decoctions because the body was not perfectly purged beforehand, or [the decoctions] were not used at an appropriate time, or the regimen was not followed carefully. Patients began to loosen up their regimen either before the viscera, damaged by the previous calamity and the appalling use of medications, recovered and regained strength, or [they started to loosen it up] immediately after their use [medicines] and did not spare the errors. This resulted in the repeated accumulation of various excrements, [pg. 682] treatment that could not be completed, and even that the fire in the matters, which were still quite susceptible to the repeated reception of its [heat], was so to say sparked again. Despite this, thanks to the careful use of that which they should have used, they were soon cured completely. A decoction of guaiacum wood in water, not in wine, which I would be concerned warms up too much, has proven more effective to me. I would recommend it [guaiacum] more because it is more favorable for the stomach than sarsaparilla, which requires a large amount, and in my opinion [guaiacum] dries out less. Because it sometimes somewhat warms one up, due to this disadvantage, I would add for each pound of [guaiacum] wood for boiling at least a handful of chicory and half a handful of borage leaves. I would boil it in such a manner in a half-covered vessel so that half remained from twelve pounds of water and one pound of sawdust or chips of [guaiacum] wood. [It is necessary] to occasionally remove the foam [and to cook it] on an even fire, such as that from lighted coal, so that the [decoction] does not expand too much. And I would also want the vessel to be carefully wrapped in a cover when it is taken off the fire and so cooled very gradually. Now, regarding the second decoction, which would be used internally. I would like it to be boiled from the same amount of water until one third boils off. From the very dawn until four in the evening before meals, may he drink eight ounces and cover himself, but adequately so that he does not get too warm and sweat. However, he must avoid the chill and not expose himself to fresh winds unless absolutely necessary. May the regimen be modest from the beginning for about ten days and then may it be even stricter. Always but with consideration of habit and with daily allowances to the level of his [the patient's] resilience. I would not want him to eat that so-called twice-baked dry bread and so dry his already dry body even more. And if he occasionally ate a meagre little piece of kid goat or [a piece of meat] from a nursing calf or young capons and chickens, I would not consider it harmful.

Index

For Product Safety Concerns and Information please contact our EU
representative GPSR@taylorandfrancis.com
Taylor & Francis Verlag GmbH, Kaufingerstraße 24, 80331 München, Germany

www.ingramcontent.com/pod-product-compliance
Ingram Content Group UK Ltd.
Pitfield, Milton Keynes, MK11 3LW, UK
UKHW022128190926
475702UK00013B/1687

9781041182672